D1235423

Biological Rhythms and Behavior

Advances in Biological Psychiatry

Vol. 11

Series Editors
J. Mendlewicz, Brussels and *H. M. van Praag,* Bronx, N.Y.

S. Karger · Basel · München · Paris · London · New York · Tokyo · Sydney

Biological Rhythms and Behavior

Volume Editors
J. Mendlewicz, Brussels, and *H. M. van Praag,* Bronx, N.Y.

53 figures and 16 tables, 1983

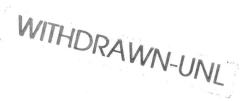

S. Karger · Basel · München · Paris · London · New York · Tokyo · Sydney

Advances in Biological Psychiatry

National Library of Medicine, Cataloging in Publication
Biological rhythms and behavior
Volume editors, J. Mendlewicz and H. M. van Praag. – Basel; New York: Karger, 1983.
(Advances in biological psychiatry; v. 11)
1. Behavior 2. Periodicity I. Praag, Herman M. van, 1929 – II. Mendlewicz, J. III. Series
W1 AD44 v. 11 [BF 637 B55 B615]
ISBN 3-8055-3672-0

Drug Dosage

The authors and the publisher have exerted every effort to ensure that drug selection and dosage set forth in this text are in accord with current recommendations and practice at the time of publication. However, in view of ongoing research, changes in government regulations, and the constant flow of information relating to drug therapy and drug reactions, the reader is urged to check the package insert for each drug for any change in indications and dosage and for added warnings and precautions. This is particularly important when the recommended agent is a new and/or infrequently employed drug.

Contents

Groos, G. A. (Bethesda, Md.): Circadian Rhythms and the Circadian System   1

Schotman, P.; Bohus, B. (Utrecht): Role of the Neuroendocrine System in Rhythms
in Brain Protein Synthesis and Behavior   10

Wirz-Justice, A. (Basel); *Wehr, T. A.* (Bethesda, Md.): Neuropsychopharmacology
and Biological Rhythms   20

Reinberg, A. (Paris); *Vieux, N.* (Petit-Couronne); *Andlauer, P.* (Annecy); *Smolensky, M.* (Houston, Tex.): Tolerance to Shift Work: A Chronobiological
Approach   35

Quabbe, H.-J.; Gregor, M.; Bumke-Vogt, C.; Witt, I.; Giannella-Neto, D. (Berlin):
Endocrine Rhythms in a Nonhuman Primate, the Rhesus Monkey   48

*Désir, D.; Van Cauter, E.; Refetoff, S.; Fang, V. S.; Golstein, J.; Fèvre-Montange,
M.; L'Hermite, M.; Robyn, C.; Jadot, C.; Szyper, M.; Spire, J.-P.; Noël, P.;
Copinschi, G.* (Brussels/Chicago, Ill./Lyon): Hormonal Changes after Jet Lag
in Normal Man   60

Lille, F.; Burnod, Y. (Paris): Professional Activity and Physiological Rhythms   64

Kripke, D. F.; Fleck, P. A.; Mullaney, D. I.; Levy, M. I. (San Diego, Calif.):
Behavioral Analogs of the REM-nonREM Cycle   72

Kalverboer, A. F. (Groningen): Neurobehavioural Organization at Early Age and
Risk for Psychopathology   80

Gjessing, L. R. (Bergen): Periodicity in 'Schizophrenia'.   95

Beersma, D. G. M.; Hoofdakker, R. H., van den; Berkestijn, H. W. B. M., van (Groningen): Circadian Rhythms in Affective Disorders. Body Temperature and
Sleep Physiology in Endogenous Depressives   114

*Mendlewicz, J.; Hoffmann, G.; Linkowski, P.; Kerkhofs, M.; Golstein, J.; Van
Haelst, L.; L'Hermite, M.; Robyn, C.; Van Cauter, E.; Weinberg, V.; Weitzman, E. D.* (Brussels): Chronobiology and Manic Depression Neuroendocrine
and Sleep EEG Parameters   128

Weitzman, E. D. (White Plains, N.Y.): Biological Rhythms in Man under Non-
Entrained Conditions and Chronotherapy for Delayed Sleep Phase Insomnia . .   136

Adv. biol. Psychiat., vol. 11, pp. 1–9 (Karger, Basel 1983)

Circadian Rhythms and the Circadian System

G. A. Groos

National Institute of Mental Health, Clinical Psychobiology Branch, Bethesda, Md., USA

It is generally recognized that circadian rhythmicity is a fundamental characteristic of virtually all physiological, biochemical and psychological functions of an organism. Circadian rhythms have been observed in animals as widely different as protozoans and primates, including man. Biological processes, ranging from mitosis to sleep, exhibit a regular daily time course with each function reaching a particular state, e. g. maximum or minimum, at a typical time of day. Figure 1 illustrates this daily fluctuation of a number of processes measured in a human subject. The illustration could be readily extended to include circadian rhythms in osmoregulation, metabolism, the production of hormones or in neurotransmitter metabolism. At the psychological level rhythms could be added in many emotional, motivational and cognitive functions. A striking fact when several rhythms within an animal or a healthy human subject are compared is the remarkably constant phase relation between each rhythm and the environmental light-dark cycle and hence between the rhythms themselves. This regularity can be generalized by the statement that bodily processes exhibit circadian organization, i. e. a temporal order in which every function is intensified during a restricted portion of the 24-hour day.

Although the concept of circadian organization is of a descriptive nature the internal temporal order of the body is assumed to reflect a purposeful strategy [1, 2]. There are three major reasons for this assumption. In the first place the vast majority of animals are faced with regular changes in the environment related to the earth's rotation. Consequently it is of adaptive significance that their physiological state is regulated in anticipation of the daily recurring variations in external conditions such as ambient temperature, humidity or illumination. The 24-hour period of the

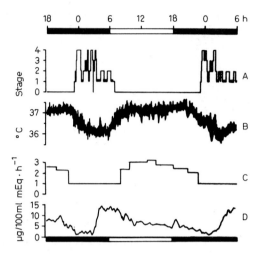

Fig. 1. Circadian rhythms recorded in a normal human subject exposed to an environmental light-dark cycle (indicated by the white and dark bars, respectively). *A* Stages of sleep (1–4) and wakefulness (0). *B* Rectal temperature rhythm. *C* Urinary potassium excretion. *D* Plasma cortisol level [*C, D* adapted from several sources, see ref. 2, 4].

earth's rotation sets a natural time base for the internal temporal order evident in the circadian system. For example, in anticipation of its diurnal activity the body temperature and metabolic rate of a bird rise even before the animal wakes up in the morning. Similarly in mammals the anticipation of food consumption will mobilize intestinal and hepatic enzymes used in the digestive process slightly before food intake is expected. Second, interdependent physiological processes can best be timed in a favorable temporal sequence. Thus, food consumption and water intake exhibit circadian rhythms with a similar time course. In man the daily diurnal efflux of potassium from the intracellular body compartment coincides with the increased renal elimination of potassium from the extracellular compartment. As a consequence the potassium concentration of the blood is maintained within a relatively narrow range during the day time. Third, the performance and stability of homeostatic control systems may be improved by the introduction of oscillatory components. Experimental support for this notion is derived from the recent finding that dissociation of circadian rhythms in thermoregulation can lead to inadequate control of body temperature in response to thermal disturbances. Thus, the presence of circadian rhythms which are appropriately timed with respect to each other

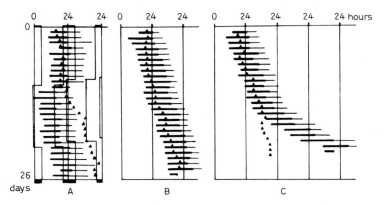

Fig. 2. The sleep-wakefulness and temperature rhythms of normal human subjects living in isolation under controlled environmental conditions. In these records the bars represent wakefulness and the lines sleep. Each complete sleep-wake cycle is plotted underneath the previous one. Subsequent experimental days are plotted vertically while the horizontal axis indicates the actual time of day. A In this experiment a subject was entrained to an artificial light-dark cycle (darkness is indicated by the dark bars at the bottom of the record). After 10 days the light-dark cycle was phase-advanced and the subject is seen to re-entrain slowly to the new regimen. The original regimen is imposed 11 days later and again re-entrainment occurs. B A stable free-run of both rhythms in constant illumination. C The subject shows internal desynchronization after 15 cycles in constant light [adapted from ref. 4].

as well as the 24-hour alternation between day and night allows for a better regulation of the internal milieu and a more efficient response to the predictable rhythmic changes in the environment.

A crucial question for the understanding of circadian organization is whether circadian rhythms are merely passive responses to the daily changes in the environment. For the majority of rhythms this is not the case [3]. If an animal or a human subject is isolated from the daily time cues and exposed to constant environmental conditions, its rhythms usually persist (fig. 2). This finding indicates that the persisting rhythms are endogenous [3, 4]. It has become customary to reserve the adjective *circadian* only to such endogenous rhythms. The endogenous nature of circadian rhythms is further demonstrated by the fact that they are innate and susceptable to genetic manipulation [5, 6]. When recorded in constant conditions, circadian rhythms develop a period which deviates somewhat from exactly 24 h [3]. In this so-called free-running state the period can be shorter or longer than 24 h depending on the experimental conditions (e. g. light intensity) or the species studied. When the circadian system of man is synchronized to the 24-hour day and subsequently allowed to free-run in constant conditions, the period of the rhythms increases to approximately 25 h. In addition, the temporal relationships between the rhythms change although eventually they remain mutually synchronized. Thus the temperature rhythm, which normally reaches its maximum a few hours before the onset of sleep and its minimum early in the morning, when it free-runs is seen to advance considerably (fig. 2). Frequently a further change occurs under these conditions. Suddenly and for no apparent reason different rhythms break away from each other and continue their free-run with different periods. The temperature rhythm may persist with a period of about 25 h while the length of the sleep-wakefulness cycle can increase to, for instance, 33 h (fig. 2). This phenomenon is known as internal desynchronization and has been documented for man and at least one non-human primate [2, 4].

The observations mentioned above, together with a number of other considerations, have led to the multioscillator model of the primate circadian system [2, 4, 7]. The model postulates that circadian rhythms are generated by multiple internal circadian pacemakers. Each rhythm is entirely or predominantly driven by a particular pacemaker and each pacemaker controls one or more rhythmic processes. The pacemakers are coupled to each other to ensure internal synchronization but, when the coupling weakens, they can run independently, each expressing its individual period. The latter phenomenon is observed in the case of internal desynchronization when different periods are measured in the overt rhythms controlled by different pacemakers. Under normal conditions the pacemakers' periods are adjusted, or entrained, to 24 h by the periodic influence of environmental time cues. The major and most reliable entraining agent is the light-dark cycle. In particular cases, however, entrainment may also result from periodic exposure to other stimuli, notably social events and the availability of food. Although the multioscillator model was originally developed for the primate circadian system, recent investigations have indicated that it may well apply to other mammals. Single oscillator alternatives have been proposed but physiological studies of circadian pacemakers lend very strong support to the multioscillator formulation.

The study of endogenous pacemakers in the mammalian circadian system started with the identification of a fiber connection from the retina to the suprachiasmatic nuclei (SCN) of the hypothalamus [8, 9]. At that time it was known that the classical visual structures in the cortex, thalamus

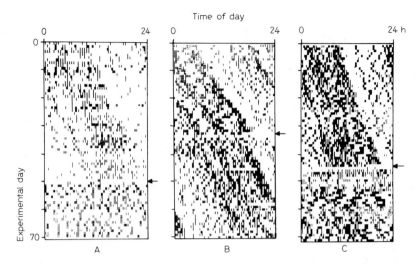

Fig. 3. Effects of lesions *(A)* and electrical *(B)* or pharmacological *(C)* stimulation of the SCN on the free-running food intake rhythm of the rat. The rhythms were recorded for over 70 consecutive experimental days. Food approaches appear as dark symbols in the records. On the days indicated by the arrows the SCN were lesioned *(A)*, electrically stimulated *(B)* or implanted with a permanently indwelling cannula with imipramine-HCl *(C)*. These procedures result in arrhythmicity *(A, C)* or a phase advance combined with a decrease in period *(B)*.

and mesencephalon were not critically involved in the entrainment of circadian rhythms to the light-dark cycle. Consequently, the discovery of the retinal projection to the SCN led to the idea that this pathway could mediate photic entrainment and that its target nucleus, the SCN, might be a circadian pacemaker. Subsequent lesion studies of the SCN confirmed these ideas [8–10]. SCN lesions in rodents as well as in the squirrel monkey result in the elimination of a wide variety of endocrine, physiological and behavioral circadian rhythms (fig. 3). At the same time lesion experiments demonstrated that the retino-hypothalamic projection to the SCN mediates the photic entrainment of circadian rhythms [9]. These lesion studies do not conclusively prove that the SCN are the substrate of a central circadian pacemaker. Several other lines of evidence, however, do support this interpretation. Destruction of SCN afferents, for instance, does not interfere with normal circadian timekeeping, while transsection of all SCN efferents results in arrhythmicity similar to that observed after SCN lesions [8]. Two completely different types of experiments provide further evidence for the pacemaker function of the SCN (fig. 3). Mild electrical stimulation and localized pharmacological stimulation of the SCN in free-running rats and hamsters have been shown to alter the most basic properties of circadian rhythms, i. e. period and phase. In addition, chronic local administration of both the monoamine oxidase inhibitor, clorgyline, and the tricyclic antidepressant, imipramine, to the SCN can cause arrhythmicity [11].

The most compelling evidence that the SCN contain a circadian pacemaker was reported by *Inouye and Kawamura* [12]. They recorded the electrical activity of the SCN and of regions elsewhere in the brain in freely moving, unanesthetized rats. While in normal animals circadian rhythms in electrical discharge can be recorded throughout the brain, only the SCN rhythm is present in animals sustaining a complete circumcision of the suprachiasmatic area. Apparently the SCN can sustain a circadian rhythm in isolation from the surrounding nervous tissue, whereas the rhythms in other brain structures seem to be driven by the SCN. In summary, there is convincing support for one of the basic assumptions of the multioscillator model of the circadian system. The identification of the SCN as a pacemaker demonstrates that endogenous circadian oscillators can indeed be found in the organism. A major question that remains is whether there is more than just one pacemaker, i. e. whether the circadian system is of a multioscillator nature.

When it was stated above that SCN lesions in mammals result in the desintegration of many circadian rhythms, it was not mentioned that there are others that persist after such a lesion. One rhythm that is not abolished by SCN lesions is the colonic temperature rhythm in the squirrel monkey [10]. While the sleep-wakefulness cycle in this primate is eliminated by a lesion of the SCN, the core temperature still shows pronounced daily oscillations both in a light-dark cycle and in constant illumination. This result not only implies the existence of a pacemaker which is located outside the SCN, but also parallels the dissociation between the sleep-wakefulness and temperature rhythms as observed during internal desynchronization in man (fig. 2). For lower mammals there is no conclusive evidence as yet for a similar differential control of these rhythms by more than one pacemaker. However, also in rodents the SCN is certainly not the only circadian pacemaker. Rodents, like many other mammals, are capable of anticipating the daily availability of food. Their rhythmic anticipatory responses to the expected meal are evident in locomotor activity, digestive enzyme mobilization and endocrine activity. The anticipation is based on a circadian timing mechanism which does not involve the SCN as SCN lesions do not affect the circadian anticipatory response to feeding schedules [13]. Unfortunately it is not known where the pacemaker of the primate temperature rhythm or the rodent anticipation cycle is located. Nevertheless, the fact of their existence is indisputable. Thus, the multioscillator model is essentially supported by the physiological investigations of the recent years.

It is justified to question whether the study of circadian rhythms is merely of interest to the biologist. Perhaps a phenomenon as pervasive and important to the functioning of the body as circadian rhythmicity has implications for psychiatry. In principle, the circadian system can be involved in mental disorders in two ways. On the one hand, an abnormal time course of circadian rhythms can be a prominent aspect of mental illness [14]. For instance, it is well known that the mood of depressed patients exhibits a pronounced daily rhythm with depression being most severe in the morning hours. On the other hand, it is possible that a disturbance within the multioscillator system contributes to mental illness as a causative factor. This idea is at the root of recent hypotheses postulating that a dissociation between rhythms controlled by different pacemakers underlie affective disorders. Rhythm abnormalities such as early phase positions of endocrine rhythms with respect to the sleep-wakefulness cycle are indeed commonly observed in manic-depressive patients. In addition changes in circadian organization can be seen in these patients when they switch from mania to depression or vice versa [14]. Such phenomena can be explained by making appropriate assumptions about the dysfunctions of the circadian system. Abnormal free-running periods, supersensitivity to the entraining light-dark cycle or weakened coupling between pacemakers are commonly proposed to account for the rhythm disturbances that accompany affective illness [14]. Unfortunately, these considerations can not serve to demonstrate a causal relation between the circadian system and the occurence of physiological and mood disturbances in mental patients. Detailed study of the formal properties of the circadian system can be helpful in this respect.

Knowledge of how the timing of rhythms can be altered by sleep deprivation, phase-shifting and other procedures will serve to establish whether the manipulation of the circadian system leads to changes in the mental state of psychiatric patients. Physiological studies can be used to investigate the effects of psychoactive drugs on identified pacemakers and consequently on the circadian system. Some initial progress has recently been made in this area [11]. This work seems of great interest as it combines the study of the possible origins of mental disorders in the circadian system with that of the action of therapeutically used compounds on the function of circumscribed parts of the nervous system, such as the suprachiasmatic nuclei.

Summary

Circadian rhythms are endogenous oscillations in physiological, biochemical and psychological functions, which are normally synchronized to the 24-hour day. They provide the body with a useful temporal organization of function. The circadian system is organized as a multioscillator structure with multiple circadian pacemakers, one of which is located in the suprachiasmatic nuclei of the brain.

References

1   Enright, J.T.: Ecological aspects of endogenous rhythmicity. Ann. Rev. ecol. Syst. *1:* 221–238 (1970).
2   Moore-Ede, M.C.; Sulzman, F.M.: Internal temporal order; in Aschoff, Handbook of behavioral neurobiology. Vol. 4: Biological rhythms, pp. 215–241 (Plenum Press, New York 1981).
3   Aschoff, J.: Circadian rhythms: influences of internal and external factors on the period measured in constant conditions. Z. Tierpsychol. *49:* 225–249 (1979).
4   Wever, R.: The circadian system of man (Springer, Berlin 1979).
5   Fuchs, J.L.; Moore, R.Y.: Development of circadian rhythmicity and light responsiveness in the rat suprachiasmatic nucleus: a study using the 2-deoxy[2–^{14}C] glucose method. Proc. natn. Acad. Sci. USA 77: 1204–1208 (1980).
6   Konopka, R.J.: Genetics and development of circadian rhythms in invertebrates; in Aschoff, Handbook of behavioral neurobiology. Vol. 4: Biological rhythms, pp. 173–181 (Plenum Press, New York, 1981).
7   Moore-Ede, M.C.; Sulzman, F.M.: The physiological basis of circadian timekeeping in primates. Physiologist, Lond. *20:* 17–25 (1977).
8   Rusak, B.; Zucker, I.: Neural regulation of circadian rhythms. Physiol. Rev. *59:* 449–526 (1979).
9   Rusak, B.: Neural mechanisms for entrainment and generation of mammalian circadian rhythms. Fed. Proc. *38:* 2589–2595 (1979).
10 Fuller, C.A.; Lydic, R.; Sulzman, F.M.; Albers, H.E.; Tepper, B.; Moore-Ede, M.C.: Circadian rhythm of body temperature persists after suprachiasmatic lesions in the squirrel monkey. Am. J. Physiol. (in press).
11 Wirz-Justice, A.; Groos, G.A.; Wehr, T.A.: The neuropharmacology of circadian timekeeping in mammals; in Aschoff, Daan, Groos, Vertebrate circadian systems: structure and physiology (Springer, Berlin, in press).

12 Inouye, S.T.; Kawamura, H.: Persistence of circadian rhythmicity in a mammalian hypothalamic island containing the suprachiasmatic nucleus. Proc. natn. Acad. Sci. USA 76: 5962–5966 (1979).
13 Stephan, F.K.: Limits of entrainment to periodic feeding in rats with suprachiasmatic lesions. J. comp. Physiol. (in press).
14 Wehr, T.A.; Goodwin, F.K.: Biological rhythms and psychiatry; in Arieti, Keith, Brody, American handbook of psychiatry, vol. 7 (Basic Books, 1981).

G.A. Groos, MD, National Institute of Mental Health, Clinical Psychobiology Branch, 9000 Rockville Pike, Bethesda, MD 20205 (USA)

Adv. biol. Psychiat., vol. 11, pp. 10–19 (Karger, Basel 1983)

Role of the Neuroendocrine System in Rhythms in Brain Protein Synthesis and Behavior

P. Schotman [a], *B. Bohus* [b, 1]

[a] Division of Molecular Neurobiology, Institute of Molecular Biology, Laboratory of Physiological Chemistry, and [b] Rudolf Magnus Institute for Pharmacology, University of Utrecht, The Netherlands

Biorhythms are fundamental features of biological systems. They are apparent in behavioral, endocrine and physiological functions. Extrinsic factors arising from the light/dark cycle, the variation of seasons and other cycles, are important determinants of rhythmicity. However, intrinsic rhythms at the level of cells and tissues appear also to exist [*Scheving* et al., 1974]. The rhythmic activities of the nervous and endocrine systems, the two main elements of regulation, interact with one another to maintain homeostasis [*Kawakami,* 1974].

During the last few years it has been established that the suprachiasmatic nucleus of the hypothalamus plays a key role in entraining circadian rhythmicity of several behavioral, endocrine and physiological functions. Destruction of the suprachiasmatic nucleus abolishes circadian rhythmicity in behavioral activity, sleep-wake cycle, adrenal corticosterone secretion, body temperature, etc. [*Moore,* 1978a]. Direct projection from the retina to the suprachiasmatic nucleus mediates information critical to the entrainment of circadian rhythmicity.

The suprachiasmatic nucleus contains parvocellular, neurosecretory nuclei that produce vasopressin [*Swaab* et al., 1975]. Vasopressinergic neurons arising from this nucleus terminate in a number of extrahypothalamic structures such as the lateral septum, the lateral habenular nuclei and dorsal thalamus [*Buijs* et al., 1978; *Buijs,* 1980]. It is therefore not unreasonable to assume that the neuropeptide vasopressin may play a

[1] Present address: Dept. of Animal Physiology, University of Groningen, Haren, The Netherlands.

role in conveying the rhythmicity message from the suprachiasmatic nucleus.

Neuropeptides, in general, seem to have an important function as mediators of behavioral changes via modulation of metabolic processes in the nervous system [*de Wied, 1977 Bohus, 1981; Gispen* et al., 1981]. For example, the central mechanism of action of ACTH and its congeners involves changes in neurotransmitter turnover, in RNA and protein synthesis, in cyclic nucleotide levels and in phosphorylation of membrane proteins and lipids [*Gispen* et al., 1981; *Dunn and Schotman*, 1981]. Discrete rhythms have been reported for the levels of several neuropeptides in specific brain regions and/or the cerebrospinal fluid [*O'Donohue* et al., 1979; *Reppert* et al., 1981].

In this article, we describe investigations on the relationship between neuropeptide levels and brain function in two model systems: (i) the influence of circadian rhythmicity in nervous activity on the modulation of pineal protein synthesis by neurohormones was studied, and (ii) the effect of changes in endogenous vasopressin levels in Brattleboro rats on the circadian variations in spontaneous activity was measured.

The pineal, or the 'third eye' has been implicated for many years as a transducer of lighting changes in the control of reproductive function. During the last few years, the pineal gland has gained considerable acceptance as a useful paradigm for the study of neuroendocrine integrative functions in general [*Axelrod*, 1974; *Nir*, 1978; *Cardinali*, 1979]. The pineal of the rat is predominantly or exclusively innervated by noradrenergic terminals arising from the superior cervical ganglion [*Moore*, 1978b]. The metabolic processes in pineal glands continue to function at physiological rates for several hours after dissection from the brain [*Wurtman* et al., 1969; *Dunlop* et al., 1977; *Schotman* et al., 1981]. Moreover, the isolated glands remain under the influence of β-noradrenergic mechanisms by virtue of the adhering noradrenergic terminals. Protein synthesis was measured during 6 h of incubation and remained at a constant rate, which was greater than 90 % of the in vivo rate [*Dunlop* et al., 1977; *Schotman* et al., 1981].

As is shown in figure 1A, the protein synthesis rate observed in vitro varied with the time the glands were dissected from the brain, being highest at midnight and lowest at 10 a.m., 2 h after the onset of light. The ratio between the peak and trough levels was about 2, which is much higher than has been observed in protein synthesis in other tissues. This may be a reflection of the lack of multiple innervation of the glands and/or an unusual high sensitivity to neural and hormonal influences. The influence of the

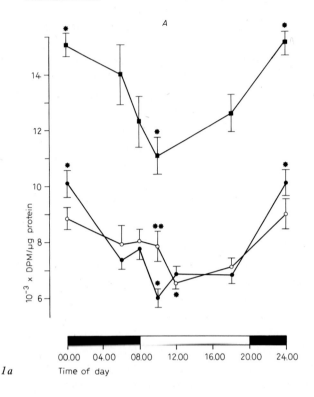

1a

Fig. 1. a Circadian rhythm. Rats were sacrificed at the times indicated on the horizontal axis and pineals were dissected. The animals were used either intact (●) or sham-operated (data not shown, not different from intact), or 5 days after decentralisation (■). Next, the incorporation of [1-^{14}C]-valine into proteins was measured under standard conditions, i.e., over a 6-hour period following 2 h of preincubation. Data from pineals of intact rats incubated in the presence of ACTH ($10^{-7}M$, O). Bars represent means $\pm$ SEM (n = 6). *p $<$ 0.01 2-way analysis of variance indicates the time points that are different from the mean obtained by averaging data over the whole day. **2p $<$ 0.05 Student's t test indicates the time points that are different as a consequence of ACTH$_{1-24}$. *b.* Dose-response curve of the sensitivity to ACTH$_{1-24}$ at 24.00 and 10.00 h. Pineals were dissected at 24.00 or 10.00 h and preincubated for 2 h. ACTH $_{1-24}$ was added at time 0 of incubation. Bars represent mean $\pm$ SEM (n = 6). *2p $<$0.01 Student's t test, ACTH vs. control.

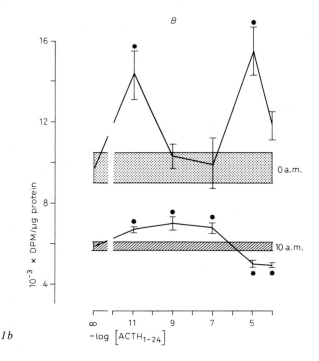

1b

CNS is clearly shown by the difference between pineals from intact rats and pineals which had been surgically decentralized 5 days prior to removal of the glands. Such deprivation of CNS input has been shown to result in a supersensitivity of the β-adrenergic receptor [*Axelrod*, 1974; *Cardinali*, 1979]. Surprisingly, the circadian rhythmicity remained. Apparently, it is not conveyed directly via the central connection as was supposed by others [*Cardinali*, 1979]. Vasopressin has been proposed as the mediator of the rhythmic influences of the suprachiasmatic nucleus on various nerve systems and it seems likely that the pineal system is under analogous neurohumoral control [*Krieger and Liotta*, 1979]. The flattening of the rhythmicity in pineal protein synthesis (fig. 1A, ○), in the presence of ACTH ($10^{-7} M$) might be an indication for the involvement of neuropeptides in the circadian variations in vivo.

The sensitivity of the pineal system to ACTH-like peptides varied over the 24-hour period in addition to the fluctuations noted above in protein synthesis (fig. 1B). The highest sensitivity was found at midnight, when the basal activity was maximal. The correlation between high basal activity and high sensitivity to hormone stimulation might be a common feature of receptor-mediated processes [*Romero and Axelrod*, 1974; *Zatz*, 1978]. The concentration-effect curve is biphasic (fig. 1); this feature has been observed in the effects of several neuropeptides on neurochemical and behavioral parameters [*Gold and van Buskirk*, 1976; *Dunn and Schotman*, 1981].

Pineal protein synthesis is also sensitive to modulation by neuropeptides other than those derived from ACTH. Desglycinamide vasopressin, a naturally occurring peptide [*de Wied*, 1977], can stimulate the synthesis rate [*Schotman* et al., 1981].

In addition to the effects of neuropeptides and of the circadian rhythms so far described in this article, pineal protein synthesis appears to be under β-noradrenergic control. The neurotransmitter norepinephrine ($10^{-6} M$), the β-agonist isoproterenol ($5 \times 10^{-9} M$) and dibutyryl cyclic AMP ($10^{-7} M$), the usual second messenger in β-adrenergic systems, stimulated pineal protein synthesis in vitro [*Schotman* et al., 1981]. Moreover, the β-antagonist propanolol ($10^{-5} M$) inhibited protein synthesis, whereas the neurotransmitters acetylcholine and dopamine were inactive. β-Noradrenergic stimulation in vitro mimics the effect of nerve input in vivo, since (i) stimulation of pineal protein synthesis by isoproterenol was observed following β-agonist administration in vivo ($5 \mu g/kg$) 1 h prior to dissection, and (ii) decentralization of the pineals rendered protein synthesis insensitive to β-noradrenergic stimulation [*Schotman* et al., 1981].

In figure 2 a scheme is presented in which the modulation of pineal protein synthesis by neurohormones, such as ACTH and vasopressin, is related to the influence of the noradrenergic innervation of the pinealocytes.

Calcium ($2 mM$) stimulates pineal protein synthesis and unlike β-noradrenergic-mediated stimulation, this calcium effect is unaltered by prior decentralization of the glands [*Schotman* et al., 1981]. Calcium also plays a role in the action of neuropeptides on the stimulation of pineal protein synthesis as shown by the dependence of this peptide effect on the presence of calcium. Calcium ions have been implicated as mediators of the effects of peptide hormones in various systems [*Farese and Prudente*, 1977; *Dunn and Schotman*, 1981]. However, an additional role for cyclic nucleotides in the neuropeptide action cannot be fully ruled out [*Dunn and Schotman*, 1981].

Thus, neurohormones, such as ACTH and vasopressin, most likely affect the pineal system in a calcium-mediated mechanism, either involving the post-synaptic β-receptor or using calcium as a second messenger.

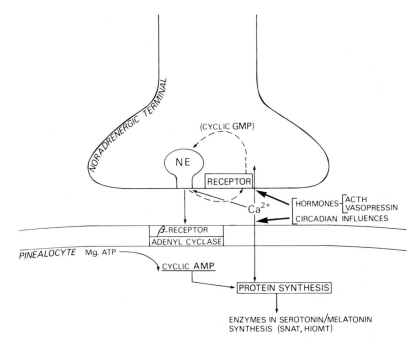

Fig. 2. Scheme for the control of pineal activity by hormonal, neural and endogenous (i.e. circadian) influences.

Circadian rhythms are maintained after decentralization (fig. 1A). This may be because they are mediated post-synaptically by calcium- and neurohormone-sensitive systems, or because they are at the level of the cervical ganglion, as has been proposed for the influence of sexual hormones [*Cardinali,* 1979].

Neurohormones seem to be as important as neural input in the mediation of circadian rhythms, as has been shown for seasonal variations [*Nir,* 1978; *Cardinali,* 1979; *Schotman* et al., 1981].

There are no data available to suggest that the modulatory influences of neuropeptides on motivational, learning and memory processes depend on circadian rhythmicity. For example, the motivational influence of ACTH-related peptides has been found in rewarded behavioral paradigms both during the light [*Garrud* et al., 1974] and the dark phase [*Bohus* et al., 1975] of the day. Similarly, vasopressin-induced facilitation of memory processes have been observed in rewarded behavioral tests during both the light [*Hostetter* et al., 1975] and the dark phase [*Bohus,* 1977]. One cannot,

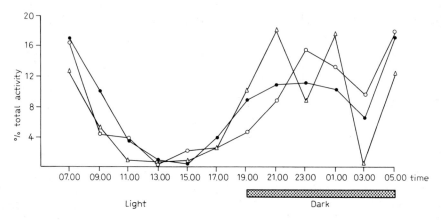

Fig. 3. Circadian activity in wheel-running activity of three variants of Brattleboro rats with differences in vasopressin synthesis and release. ○ = Diabetes insipidus; △ = heterozygous; ● = normal.

however, exclude the possibility that the sensitivity of the behavioral measures that were used in the above-mentioned studies are not sufficient to demonstrate given differences in the sensitivity of rats to neuropeptide treatment.

More spontaneous behavioral activities, such as locomotion, exploratory behavior, wheel-running activity of the rat show clear-cut circadian variations in relation to the light-dark cycle. These behavioral activities of the rat and other rodents are higher in the dark than in light. In order to investigate the possibility that vasopressin is an intermediator of the influence of the CNS on rhythmicity, the behavioral rhythmicity of Brattleboro rats has been studied.

A homozygous variant of the Brattleboro strain lacks the ability to synthesize vasopressin due to a single gene deficit and suffers hypothalamic diabetes insipidus. Heterozygous variants of this strain display disturbed synthesis and release of vasopressin [*Valtin and Schroeder,* 1964]. If vasopressin plays an essential role in circadian rhythmicity of behavioral activities, one might expect that rhythmicity would be absent in these rats. However, the homozygous diabetes insipidus rats exhibit normal diurnal rhythmicity in wheel-running activity (fig. 3). The daily pattern of the activity of the diabetes insipidus rats (dark peak and light trough) was comparable to that of the normal variant of this strain. Thus, the absence of vasopressin is not associated with the absence of behavioral rhythmicity.

Heterozygous Brattleboro rats also exhibited rhythmicity with more activity in the dark and less in the light period (fig. 3). It is, however, remarkable that the activity curve of the heterozygous rats showed large variations during the dark phase in contrast to homozygous diabetes insipidus and normal Brattleboro rats. These observations suggest that the diabetic rats may be able to adapt to the complete absence of vasopressin. However, if vasopressin release is only impaired, as is the case in heterozygous rats, a given modulation of rhythmic behavior is disturbed.

Gold et al. [1978] launched the hypothesis that vasopressin may play a role in disorders of human behavior, in particular in manic-depressive illness. Disturbances of rhythmicity in endocrine, sleep-wake, etc., functions are prominent features of manic-depressive illness. Cognitive deficits can also be observed. Animal experiments led to the conclusion that vasopressin plays an important role in memory and cognition [de Wied, 1977; Bohus, 1981]. Vasopressin treatment enhances cognitive function in depressive patients while other symptoms are frequently not ameliorated by the neuropeptides [Gold et al., 1980]. This is compatible with the experimental findings, i.e., vasopressin plays a more essential role in the modulation of memory and cognition than in behavioral rhythmicity.

In conclusion, neuropeptides and neurohormones are implicated as important modulators of metabolic processes in the CNS [Gispen et al., 1981]. Their levels in the CNS show distinct circadian rhythmicity [Kawakami, 1974; O'Donohue et al., 1979; Reppert et al., 1981].

In the pineal, neuropeptides may act as mediators of centrally evoked rhythmic changes in protein synthesis [Nir, 1978; Schotman et al., 1981], resulting in changes in enzyme activities [Wurtman et al., 1969].

β-Noradrenergic receptor systems have been proposed for the regulation of metabolic processes in the pineal [Axelrod, 1974]. In addition, neurohormones seem to be involved using Ca^{2+}-mediated processes.

Although neuropeptides and neurohormones have been implicated in the control of several behavioral processes in rodents and man [de Wied, 1977; Gold et al., 1980; Bohus, 1981], the data concerning their influences on circadian rhythmicity in behavior are still scarce.

Summary

Neuroendocrine rhythms may be mediators of rhythmic changes in brain protein synthesis and behavior. Congeners of ACTH and vasopressin are candidates for such a modulatory role. The pineal gland, which may serve as a model for the brain, shows marked circadian variations in protein synthesis and in the sensitivity of protein synthesis to neuropeptides. β-Noradrenergic mechanisms appear to be involved in the circadian variations.

Behavioral abnormalities in two strains of Brattleboro rat displaying disturbed vasopressin synthesis were restricted to irregularities in spontaneous behavior. Nevertheless, there are strong indications that vasopressin plays an important role in memory and cognition. In depressed patients, vasopressin is able to enhance the disturbed cognitive function specifically.

Acknowledgements

We greatly acknowledge Prof. Dr. *W. H. Gispen* and Dr. *P. Edwards* for their most valuable discussions on the subject of this article, and Mr. *E. Kluis* and Miss *L. Claessens* for their technical assistance with the preparation of this manuscript.

Part of this research was supported by the Netherlands Organization for the Advancement of Pure Research.

References

Axelrod, J.: The pineal gland: a neurochemical transducer. Science *184:* 1341–1348 (1974).

Bohus, B.: Effect of desglycinamide lysine vasopressin (DG-LVP) on sexually motivated T-maze behavior of the male rat. Horm. Behav. *8:* 52–61 (1977).

Bohus, B.: Neuropeptides in brain functions and dysfunctions. Int. J. ment. Health *9:* 6–44 (1981).

Bohus, B.; Hendrikx, H. H. L.; Kolfschoten, A. A. van; Krediet, T. G.: The effect of ACTH$_{4-10}$ on copulatory and sexually motivated approach behavior in the male rat; in Sandler, Gessa, Sexual behavior: pharmacology and biochemistry, pp. 269–275 (Raven Press, New York 1975).

Buijs, R. M.: Intra- and extrahypothalamic vasopressin and oxytocin pathways in the rat. Pathways to the limbic system, medulla oblongata and spinal cord. Cell Tiss. Res. *192:* 423–435 (1980).

Buijs R. M.; Swaab, D. F.; Dogterom, J.; Leuven, F. V. van: Intra- and extrahypothalamic vasopressin and oxytocin pathways in the rat. Cell Tiss. Res. *186:* 423–433 (1978).

Cardinali, D. P.: Models in neuroendocrinology. Neurohumoral pathways to the pineal gland. Trends Neurosci. *2:* 250–253 (1979).

Dunlop, D. S.; Elden, W. van; Lajtha, A.: Developmental effects on protein synthesis rates in regions of the CNS in vivo and in vitro. J. Neurochem. *29:* 939–945 (1977).

Dunn, A. J.; Schotman, P.: Effects of ACTH and related peptides on RNA and protein synthesis. J. Pharmac. exp. Ther. *12:* 353–372 (1981).

Farese, R. V.; Prudente, W. J.: Localization of the metabolic processes affected by calcium during corticotropin action. Biochim. biophys. Acta *497:* 386–395 (1977).

Garrud, P.; Gray, J. A.; Wied, D. de: Pituitary-adrenal hormones and extinction of rewarded behaviour in the rat. Physiol. Behav. *12:* 109–119 (1974).

Gispen, W. H.; Someren, H. van, Schotman, P.: Molecular aspects of ACTH-brain interaction. Adv. Physiol. Sci. *13:* 223–231 (1981).

Gold, P. E.; Buskirk, R. B. van: Enhancement and impairment of memory processes with post-trial injections of adrenocorticotrophic hormone. Behav. Biol. *16:* 387–400 (1976).

Gold, P. W.; Goodwin, F. K.; Ballenger, J. C.; Weingartner, H.; Robertson, G. L.; Post, R. N.: Central vasopressin function in affective illness; in De Wied, van Keep, Hormones and the brain, pp. 241–252 (MTP Press, Lancaster 1980).

Gold, P. W.; Goodwin, E. K.; Reus, V. I.: Vasopressin in affective illness. Lancet *i:* 1233–1236 (1978).

Hostetter, G.; Jupp, S. L.; Kozlowski, G. P.: Vasopressin affects the behavior of rats in a positively-rewarded discrimination task. Life Sci. *21:* 1323–1328 (1975).

Kawakami, M.: Biological rhythms in neuroendocrine activity (Igaku Shoin, Tokyo 1974).

Krieger, D. T.; Liotta, A. S.: Pituitary hormones in brain: where, how, and why? Science *205:* 366–371 (1979).

Moore, R. Y.: Central neural control of circadian rhythms. Front. Neuroendocrinol., vol. 5, pp. 185–206 (Raven Press, New York 1978a).

Moore, R. Y.: Neural control of pineal function in mammals and birds. J. neural Transm., suppl. 13, pp. 47–58 (1978b).

Nir, I.: Non-reproductive systems and the pineal gland. J. neural Transm., suppl. 13, pp. 225–244 (1978).

O'Donohue, T. L.; Miller, R. L.; Pendleton, R. C.; Jacobowitz, D. M.: A diurnal rhythm of α-melanocyte-stimulating hormone in discrete regions of the rat brain. Neuroendocrinology *29:* 281–287 (1979).

Reppert, S. M.; Artman, H. G.; Swaminathan, S.; Fisher, D. A.: Vasopressin exhibits a rhythmic daily pattern in cerebrospinal fluid but not in blood. Science *213:* 1256–1257 (1981).

Romero, J. A.; Axelrod, J.: Pineal beta-adrenergic receptor: diurnal variations in sensitivity. Science *184:* 1091–1092 (1974).

Scheving, L. E.; Halberg, F.; Pauly, J. E.: Chronobiology (Thieme, Stuttgart 1974).

Schotman, P.; Allaart, J.; Gispen, W. H.: Pineal protein synthesis highly sensitive to ACTH-like neuropeptides. Brain Res. *219:* 121–135 (1981).

Swaab, D. F.; Pool, C. W.; Nijveldt, F.: Immunofluorescence of vasopressin and oxytocin in the rat hypothalamo-neurohypophyseal system. J. neural Transm. *36:* 195–215 (1975).

Valtin, H.; Schroeder, H. A.: Familiar hypothalamic diabetes insipidus in rats (Brattleboro). Am. J. Physiol. *206:* 425–430 (1964).

Wied, D. de: Minireview: peptides and behavior. Life Sci. *20:* 195–204 (1977).

Wurtman, R. J.; Stein, H. M.; Axelrod, J.; Larin, F.: Incorporation of ^{14}C-tryptophan into ^{14}C-protein by cultured rat pineal: stimulation by L-norepinephrine. Proc. natn. Acad. Sci. USA *62:* 749–755 (1969).

Zatz, M.: Sensitivity and cyclic nucleotides in the rat pineal gland. J. neural Transm., suppl. 13, pp. 175–201 (1978).

Dr. P. Schotman, Institute of Molecular Biology, State University of Utrecht, P. O. Box 80.063, NL-3508 TB Utrecht (The Netherlands)

Adv. biol. Psychiat., vol. 11, pp. 20–34 (Karger, Basel 1983)

Neuropsychopharmacology and Biological Rhythms

Anna Wirz-Justice[1], *Thomas A. Wehr*

Clinical Psychobiology Branch, National Institute of Mental Health,
Bethesda, Md., USA

Introduction

Why should we look at the effects of psychoactive drugs on biological rhythms? What information can be gained from looking at biochemistry and behavior in terms of a system rather than any single component? How can the neuropsychopharmacology of biological rhythms provide information as to mechanisms? And what is the therapeutic consequence of such an integration of disciplines?

This paper summarises basic and experimental studies using a new conceptual approach (but old methods) to neuropsychopharmacology that has arisen primarily from clinical studies. It is no new observation that affective illness is characterized by marked periodic manifestations: diurnal variation of symptom severity, early morning awakening, hormonal and seasonal exacerbations, and the cyclicity of the illness itself.

'In the true endogenous depressive we see a shift in the 24-hour rhythm, a phase shift that can express itself from a slight phase shift to a complete reversal – the night becomes day. Anyone knowing the material would look for the CNS origin in the midbrain, where the entire vegetative nervous system is controlled by a central clock whose rhythmicity ... regulates and balances the biological system' *Georgi* [1947].

Since this remarkably astute analysis, 30 years of clinical research have brought little information in terms of biological rhythms. It was only in 1975 when *Papousek* elegantly formulated a precise hypothesis in terms of sleep disturbances found in depression that a renewed interest in these phenomena arose:

---

[1] Visiting Fellow of the Schweizerische Stiftung für medizinisch-biologische Stipendien.

'Somnopathy in depressive patients is based on an internal and external desynchronisation ... the reduced REM latency, the relative increase in REM sleep at the beginning of the night, and the shortening of REM cycles ... find a new interpretation as the expression of a phase displacement of the circadian rhythm of REM activity' *Papousek* [1975].

Two further advances were important. First, elucidation of the formal properties of the human circadian system in the pioneering studies of *Aschoff* [1982] and *Wever* [1979] provided a normal physiology of biological rhythms and a model. Second, delineation of a potential morphological substrate for the 'biological clock' in mammals (including man), in the suprachiasmatic nuclei of the anterior hypothalamus [for review, see *Groos,* this volume], provided a time base and drive for the complex daily cycle of physiological and behavioral events. This knowledge of a neuroanatomical locus for circadian timekeeping and its functional correlates was a necessary prerequisite for any model of circadian pathophysiology.

Circadian Rhythm Phase Advance Hypothesis of Depression

The human circadian system has been modelled by two endogenous, self-sustained, coupled oscillators: a strong one controlling body temperature, REM-sleep propensity and cortisol secretion, and a weak one controlling the sleep-wake cycle and sleep-related neuroendocrine activity [*Wever,* 1979][2]. Normally, the coupled oscillator system is entrained to the 24-hour day; however, the phase-relationships between the two oscillators can be temporarily disturbed (e. g. by transmeridian travel) and can spontaneously dissociate under conditions of isolation from external time cues [*Wever,* 1979]. There are several ways in which such a homeostatically controlled system could be altered by disease or by treatment interventions [*Wehr* et al., 1982b; *Aschoff,* 1982]. These changes (in frequency, amplitude, and/or coupling) could be expected to affect the phase-position of circadian rhythms entrained to the day-night cycle. There is scattered and indirect experimental evidence that the sleep and neuroendocrine abnormalities observed in depressive patients may be a consequence or correlate of a phase advance of the circadian oscillator driving REM sleep propensity, temperature, and cortisol, with respect to the sleep-wake or

[2] There is also a multi-oscillator model of the sleep-wake cycle [*Enright,* 1980], and a single-oscillator model [*Eastman,* 1982], combined with a homeostatic regulatory process of sleep and wakefulness [*Borbély,* 1982; *Daan and Beersma,* 1982].

day-night cycle. We have elsewhere analyzed the available data in the literature [*Wehr and Goodwin*, 1981] and found a remarkably consistent phase advance of many circadian rhythms in depressed patients. We have also carried out a preliminary clinical test of the hypothesis by phase advancing the sleep-wake cycle with concomitant remission of depressive symptomatology and normalization of sleep architecture [*Wehr* et al., 1979; *Wehr and Wirz-Justice*, 1981]. However, another approach to testing the hypothesis that this phase advance of circadian rhythms is pathognomonic, is to experimentally measure the effects of modalities that have empirically been found to be antidepressant on the circadian system.

Circadian Rhythm Phase Delay Hypothesis of Antidepressant Drug Action

The circadian rhythm phase advance hypothesis predicts that clinically effective antidepressant drugs should delay the phase position of circadian rhythms under entrained conditions [*Wehr* et al., 1982b]. Furthermore, in order to interpret a phase delay of an overt rhythm in terms of the underlying oscillator, the free-running circadian period (τ, the duration of one complete cycle in an environment free of time cues) is the only parameter that reflects the frequency of the oscillator [*Pittendrigh and Daan*, 1976]. The classic studies in both man and rodents on the properties of circadian pacemakers have measured the free-running period of the rest-activity cycle. Until now, only very few substances have been found that can modify frequency in mammals: the endogenously occurring hormones (estradiol, testosterone, thyroid), heavy water and carbachol [for reviews see *Turek and Gwinner*, 1982; *Wirz-Justice* et al., 1982b]. τ is homeostatically conserved [*Richter*, 1965, *Pittendrigh and Caldarola*, 1973]. It is therefore of some significance that three neuropharmacologically active substances (all used in the treatment of affective disorders) have recently been shown to modify frequency and phase position of circadian rhythms.

Lithium

Lithium is used as an antimanic agent and prophylactic drug for recurrent affective illness. It was the first psychoactive drug investigated in terms of its effect on circadian rhythms, and has been the most extensively

Table I. Effect of lithium on free-running circadian rhythms

Species	Rhythm parameter	Effect	Reference
Desert cactus	petal opening in constant green light	lengthens τ dose-response curve	*Engelmann* [1973]
Cockroach	rest-activity cycle in constant dim red light	lengthens τ	*Hofmann* et al. [1978]
Aplysia	compound action potentials in isolated eye in DD	lengthens τ dose-response curve	*Strumwasser and Viele* [1980]
Hamster	rest-activity cycle in constant dim red light	lengthens τ	*Hofmann* et al. [1978] *Engelmann* [unpublished observations]
Hamster	rest-activity cycle in constant dim white light	lengthens τ	*Zucker* [unpublished observations]
Desert rat	rest-activity cycle in constant dim red light	lengthens τ	*Engelmann* [1973]
Rat	rest-activity cycle in blinded animals	lengthens τ	*Kripke and Wyborney* [1980]
Rat	feeding rhythm in blinded animals	lengthens τ	*Groos* [unpublished observations]
Man	rest-activity cycle in temperature rhythm in Arctic summer (LL)	lengthens τ	*Johnsson* et al. [1979, 1980]

studied. Lithium slows free-running rhythms in many species, including man (table I). Lithium also appears to alter the range of entrainment towards longer days [*McEachron* et al., 1981]. Furthermore, lithium delays the phase position of the sleep-wake cycle under entrained conditions [*Kripke* et al., 1979]. There are two recent studies on phase position in rodents: lithium delays many neuroendocrine, plasma electrolyte [*McEachron* et al., 1982] and CNS neurotransmitter receptor rhythms [*Kafka* et al., 1982] (examples in figure 2, summary in table II). Thus the evidence for the lithium ion's capacity to slow circadian rhythms is substantial. Clinical studies also suggest that lithium can slow or delay circadian rhythms in manic-depressive patients [*Kripke* et al., 1978].

A Monoamine Oxidase Inhibitor

The monoamine oxidase inhibitor (MAO-I) clorgyline belongs to the second generation of this class of drugs. Clinically, clorgyline is an effective

Table II. Effects of antidepressant modalities on receptor rhythm parameters

Receptor	Phase position[1]					Amplitude[2]					24-hour mean				
	imipramine	clorgyline	sleep deprivation	lithium	flu-phenazine	imipramine	clorgyline	sleep deprivation	lithium	flu-phenazine	imipramine	clorgyline	sleep deprivation	lithium	flu-phenazine
Alpha-adrenergic	-	-	-	×	-	◇	=	◇	◇	◇	◇	=	=	◆	◆
Beta-adrenergic	-	-	0	×	-	◇	=	◇	◇	=	◆	=	=	◆	◆
Benzodiazepine	0	-	0	×	-	◇	=	◇	◇	=	=	=	=	◇	=
Opiate	-	?	0	-	-	◇	◇	=	◇	◇	◆	=	=	◆	◆
Muscarinic cholinergic	?	?	0	-	?	=	◇	◇	◇	◇	◇	◆	=	◆	◆
Striatal dopamine	-	×	0	?	?	◇	=	◇	=	◇	◇	◆	=	◆	◆
Striatal benzodiazepine	-	-	-	-	×	◇	=	◇	=	=	=	◆	=	◇	◆

[1] Estimated by cosine fit to mean at each time point: - = peak later; 0 = no change; × = no rhythm; ? = change in wave form.
[2] Estimated by △ peak:trough >15%; = = no change.
◇ = p < 0.01; ◆ = p < 0.001; = = no change.

antidepressant [*Lipper* et al., 1979] and has also been observed to induce switches out of depression into hypomania, a characteristic shared with other MAO-Is [*Wehr and Goodwin,* 1979]. We have investigated this drug for its effects on τ, phase position of the rest-activity cycle and, in order to link the circadian aspect to present neuropharmacological strategies, on phase position of neurotransmitter receptor rhythms. Clorgyline was found to slow the free-running rhythm in hamsters and delay onset of nocturnal activity in a dose-dependent manner [*Wirz-Justice and Campbell,* 1982; *Wirz-Justice* et al., 1982b; *Wehr* et al., 1982b]. In addition (and in contrast to lithium), clorgyline also induced dissociation of circadian activity components [*Wirz-Justice and Wehr,* 1981; *Wirz-Justice and Campbell,* 1982] (fig. 1). In terms of biochemical rhythms, clorgyline was found to delay the phase-position of many neurotransmitter receptor rhythms [*Wirz-Justice* et al., 1982a] (examples in fig. 2). In this respect, the ability of clorgyline to down-regulate adrenergic receptor number [*Cohen* et al., 1982] was extended to include the temporal dimension. The complexity of drug effects is illustrated by a summary of chronic clorgyline modulation of the rhythm parameters of wave form, amplitude, 24-hour mean and phase (table II).

In a further experiment to investigate whether clorgyline exerts its effects on circadian rhythms directly through its action on the putative central oscillator, the suprachiasmatic nuclei (SCN), the drug was chronically applied directly to the suprachiasmatic region [*Groos and Mason,* 1982; *Wirz-Justice* et al., 1982b]. The free-running rhythms of food intake were abolished or, with lower doses, τ was lengthened. Clorgyline administration lateral or dorsal to the SCN, or empty cannulas in the SCN, did not modify rhythmicity in any respect. These findings support the hypothesis that clorgyline modifies circadian rhythm parameters by pharmacological modulation of pacemaker frequency in the SCN rather than by diffuse action on a number of brain structures.

A Tricyclic Antidepressant

The tricyclic antidepressant, imipramine, is still the classic thymoleptic drug. It can also induce switches out of depression into hypomania [*Wehr and Goodwin,* 1979]. A series of studies, similar to those carried out with clorgyline, gave analogous but less conclusive results: imipramine was found to slow the free-running rest-activity cycle in a few animals (fig. 1), but tended rather to induce dissociation of activity components [*Wirz-Justice and Campbell,* 1982; *Wirz-Justice* et al., 1982b; *Wirz-Justice and Wehr,* 1981] and delay the phase-position of many neurotransmitter receptor rhythms [*Wirz-Justice* et al., 1980; *Naber* et al., 1980; *Kafka* et al., 1981b] (examples in fig. 3, summary in table II). Implanted in the SCN, free-running rhythms were consistently abolished by imipramine [*Groos and Mason,* 1982; *Wirz-Justice* et al., 1982b]. Thus two classes of antidepressant drugs appear to have direct effects on the frequency of the

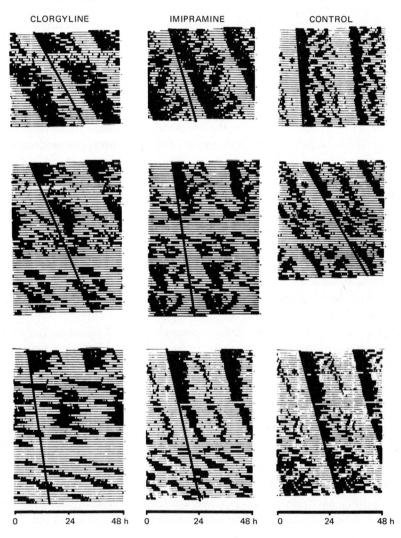

CLORGYLINE   IMIPRAMINE   CONTROL

0   24   48 h   0   24   48 h   0   24   48 h

circadian pacemaker, as reflected by the lengthened period and delayed phase position of measured rhythms.

Sleep Deprivation

A single night's sleep deprivation has been found to lead to rapid amelioration of depressive symptomatology: it has been proposed that the therapeutic effect results from modification of circadian rhythms [*Pflug and Tölle*, 1971; *Papousek*, 1975]. In order to compare sleep deprivation with chronic antidepressants, in terms of the present hypothesis, the effect of sleep deprivation on τ was measured, as well as the phase position of neurotransmitter receptor rhythms. Sleep deprivation had no effect on the period of the circadian rest-activity cycle [*Borbély and Tobler*, unpublished data], nor did it modify the phase position of receptor rhythms [*Wirz-Justice* et al., 1981] (fig. 3; table II). This contrast with respect to chronic antidepressant drugs may be related to the clinical differences in therapeutic response (acute vs. chronic) and indicates that sleep deprivation does not act through the circadian system per se [*Wehr and Wirz-Justice*, 1981].

Specificity and Therapeutic Implications

These experiments with clorgyline and imipramine, together with earlier studies with lithium, provide substantial evidence that antidepres-

---

Fig. 1. Representative running-wheel activity records of female hamsters free-running in constant dim red light. Each actogram is double plotted to permit visualization of the circadian rhythm. The period of the free-running rhythm before implantation is indicated by the vertical lines fitted to activity onset. On the days indicated by an asterisk, the animals were implanted subcutaneously with osmotic minipumps containing solutions of clorgyline (administered at 2 mg/kg/day, for at least 2 weeks), imipramine (20 mg/kg/day, for at least 2 weeks), or empty (controls). The upper actograms show hamsters whose coupled rest-activity cycle was lenghtened by both drugs. The middle actograms show a preferential lengthening of the late or morning activity component which crosses the rest phase and shows relative coordination with the early or evening activity component. The lower actograms show two extreme phenomena: with clorgyline, marked lengthening of τ occurs and the rest-activity cycle appears to break away from and show relative coordination with an underlying shorter circadian component; with imipramine, τ first lengthens, but the rest-activity cycle later shows splitting of activity components, both of which appear to undergo relative coordination with an underlying shorter circadian component [discussed in detail in *Wirz-Justice and Wehr*, 1980].

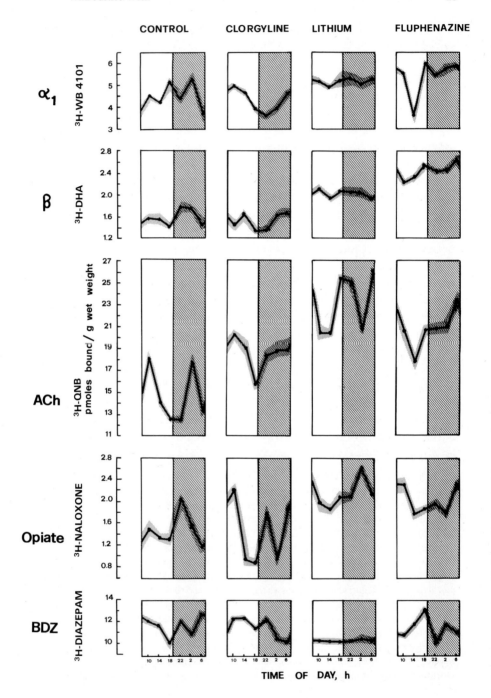

CONTROL   CLORGYLINE   LITHIUM   FLUPHENAZINE

α₁   ³H-WB 4101

β   ³H-DHA

ACh   ³H-QNB pmoles bound / g wet weight

Opiate   ³H-NALOXONE

BDZ   ³H-DIAZEPAM

TIME   OF   DAY, h

sant drugs modulate the frequency of circadian oscillations. The question of specificity is still open: do all clinically effective antidepressants slow circadian rhythms? Is this a characteristic only of antidepressants or of a wider group of psychoactive drugs? One experiment with the neuroleptic fluphenazine indicates that this drug can also delay the phase position of neurotransmitter receptors [*Naber* et al., 1982] (fig. 2; table II). Further studies will show whether the number of drugs that can modulate frequency is larger than that envisaged by *Richter* [1965] and *Pittendrigh and Caldarola* [1973] in their statements on the need for temporal invariance despite chemical fluctuations in the internal milieu. However, if psychoactive drugs prove to be powerful modulators of frequency, their mechanisms of action may be better understood in terms of a 'psychopharmacology of phase' than in the present paradigm of 'up- and down-regulation'.

This review of the present knowledge of antidepressant drug action within a circadian hypothesis of affective disorders is not without implications for therapy. New approaches to treatment and drug screening involve direct manipulation of the circadian system and/or the sleep-wake (rest-activity) cycle. One step in this direction has already been made. Strong light alone – in man high intensity is necessary [*Lewy* et al., 1980] – can, when given at the right time(s) of day, act as an antidepressant [*Lewy* et al., 1982]. Both tricyclics and MAO-Is can, in bipolar depressive patients, precipitate mania and even lead to rapid cycling between depression and mania [*Wehr and Goodwin*, 1979; *Kukopulos* et al., 1980], whereas lithium rarely has this effect. Both tricyclics and MAO-I can, in the animal model, induce dissociation of circadian activity components that may be analogous to the switch into mania [*Wehr* et al., 1982a], whereas lithium does not appear to do this [*Groos, Engelmann,* personal commun]. Thus theoretical considerations as well as clinical observations suggest that it may be necessary to withhold conventional antidepressant treatment from rapidly

---

Fig. 2. Circadian rhythms of binding of ^{3}H-WB4101 to the α_1-adrenergic receptor, ^{3}H-dihydroalprenolol to the β-adrenergic receptor, ^{3}H-quinuclidinyl benzylate to the muscarinic cholinergic receptor, ^{3}H-naloxone to the opiate receptor, and ^{3}H-diazepam to the benzodiazepine receptor in forebrain homogenates [experimental details in *Kafka* et al., 1981 a, b; *Naber* et al., 1980, 1981; *Marangos* et al., 1979]. Binding of ligands in control animals is compared with that in rats chronically treated with: clorgyline, 2 mg/kg/day for 2 weeks; lithium carbonate in chow containing 0.06 % by weight for 2 weeks; fluphenazine, 3 × weekly depot injections of 10 mg/kg. The experiment was carried out in October 1979 (n = 7 animals at each time point; mean ± s.e.m. as shaded outline). The dark phase from 19 to 7h is indicated by the hatched portion of the graph.

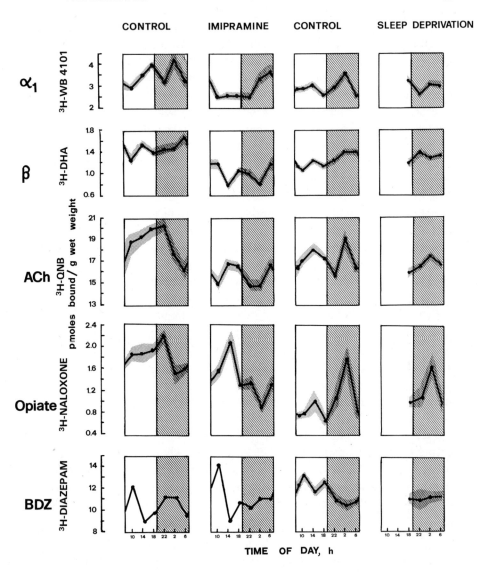

Fig. 3. Circadian rhythms of receptor binding as detailed in fig. 2. The left-hand experiment compares controls with imipramine-treated animals (10 mg/kg/day i.p. for 3 weeks), carried out in June, 1979 (n = 7 at each time point). The right-hand experiment compares controls with animals who have been deprived of sleep from the beginning of the light phase for 11–23 h, carried out in December 1979–January 1980 (n = 6 at each time point).

cycling manic-depressive patients, in spite of compelling pressures to administer them. Many of these patients may ultimately improve if lithium alone is administered [*Wehr and Goodwin*, 1979].

Experimental studies on the neuropharmacology of circadian timekeeping arose from clinical observations. In turn, these animal studies have prompted new treatment modalities that indicate more similarities between clorgyline, imipramine and lithium (slowing the circadian pacemaker) than differences (induction rather than prevention of manic states). Very low dosage regimens of clorgyline have been found to be an effective prophylactic agent in rapidly cycling manic-depressive patients who did not respond to lithium alone [*Potter* et al., 1982].

The field of circadian neuropharmacology is new. The methodology is not easy. We do, however, consider that further exploration will yield insights into basic mechanisms of action of psychoactive drugs as well as new therapies.

Acknowledgements

The active collaboration of M. S. Kafka, D. Naber, P. J. Marangos and I. C. Campbell was indispensable for these studies.

References

Aschoff, J.: Disorders of the circadian system as discussed in psychiatric research; in Wehr, Goodwin, Circadian rhythms in psychiatry. Neuroscience Series (Boxwood Press, Los Angeles 1982).

Borbély, A. A.: A two process model of sleep regulation. Hum. Neurobiol. *1:* 195–204 (1982).

Cohen, R. M.; Campbell, I. C.; Dauphin, M.; Tallman, J. F.; Murphy, D. L.: Changes in α- and β-receptor densities in rat brain as a result of treatment with monoamine oxidase inhibiting (MAOI) antidepressants. Neuropharmacology *21:* 293–298 (1982).

Daan, S.; Beersma, D.: Circadian gating of human sleep and wakefulness; in Moore-Ede, Czeisler, Mathematical modeling of circadian systems (Raven Press, New York 1982).

Eastman, C.: Are separate 'temperature' and 'activity' oscillators necessary to explain the phenomena of human circadian rhythms?; in Moore-Ede, Czeisler, Mathematical modeling of circadian systems (Raven Press, New York 1982).

Engelmann, W.: A slowing down of circadian rhythms by lithium ions. Z. Naturf. *28c:* 733–736 (1973).

Enright, J. T.: The timing of sleep and wakefulness. On the substructure and dynamics of the circadian pacemakers underlying the wake-sleep cycle (Springer, Berlin 1980).

Georgi, F.: Psychiatrische Probleme im Lichte der Rhythmusforschung. Schweiz. Med. Wschr. *49:* 1276–1280 (1947).

Groos, G. A.; Mason, R.: An electrophysiological study of the rat's suprachiasmatic nucleus: a locus for the action of antidepressants. J. Physiol., Lond. *330:* 40 (1982).

Hofmann, K.; Günderoth-Palmowski, M.; Wiedenmann, G.; Engelmann, W.: Further evidence for period lengthening effect of Li⁺ on circadian rhythms. Z. Naturf. *32c:* 231–234 (1978).

Johnsson, A.; Engelmann, W.; Pflug, B.; Klemke, W.: Influence of lithium ions on human circadian rhythms. Z. Naturf. *35c:* 503–507 (1980).

Johnsson, A.; Pflug, B.; Engelmann, W.; Klemke, W.: Effect of lithium carbonate on circadian periodicity in humans. Pharmacopsychiatria *12:* 423–425 (1979).

Kafka, M. S.; Wirz-Justice, A.; Naber, D.: Circadian and seasonal rhythms in α- and β-adrenergic receptors in the rat brain. Brain Res. *207:* 409–419 (1981a).

Kafka, M. S.; Wirz-Justice, A.; Naber, D.; Marangos, P. J.; O'Donohue, T. L.; Wehr, T. A.: The effect of lithium on circadian neurotransmitter receptor rhythms. Neuropsychobiology *8:* 41–50 (1982).

Kafka, M. S.; Wirz-Justice, A.; Naber, D.; Wehr, T. A.: Circadian acetylcholine receptor rhythm in rat brain and its modification by imipramine. Neuropharmacology *20:* 421–425 (1981b).

Kripke, D. F.; Judd, L. L.; Hubbard, B.; Janowsky, D. S.; Huey, L. Y.: The effect of lithium carbonate on the circadian rhythm of sleep in normal human subjects. Biol. Psychiat. *14:* 545–548 (1979).

Kripke, D. F.; Mullaney, D. J.; Atkinson, M.; Wolf, S.: Circadian rhythm disorders in manic-depressives. Biol. Psychiat. *13:* 335–351 (1978).

Kripke, D. F.; Wyborney, V. G.: Lithium slows rat circadian activity rhythms. Life Sci. *26:* 1319–1321 (1980).

Kukopulos, A.; Reginaldi, D.; Laddomada, P.; Floris, G.; Serra, G.; Tondo, L.: Course of the manic-depressive cycle and changes caused by treatments. Pharmacopsychiatria *13:* 156–163 (1980).

Lewy, A. J.; Wehr, T. A.; Goodwin, F. K.; Newsome, D. A.; Markey, S. P.: Light suppresses melatonin secretion in man. Science *210:* 1267–1269 (1980).

Lewy, A. J.; Kern, H. A.; Rosenthal, N. E.; Wehr, T. A.: Bright artificial light treatment of a manic-depressive patient with a seasonable mood cycle. Am. J. Psychiat. *139:* 1496–1498 (1982).

Lipper, S.; Murphy, D. L.; Slater, S.; Buchsbaum, M. S.: Comparative behavioural effects of clorgyline and pargyline in man: a preliminary evaluation. Psychopharmacology *62:* 123–128 (1979).

Marangos, P. J.; Paul, S. M.; Parma, A. M.; Goodwin, F. K.; Syapin, P.; Skolnick, P.: Purinergic inhibition of diazepam binding to rat brain (in vitro). Life Sci. *24:* 851–858 (1979).

McEachron, D. L.; Kripke, D. F.; Hawkins, R.; Haus, E.; Pavlinac, D.; Deftos, L.: Lithium delays biochemical circadian rhythms in rats. Neuropsychobiology *8:* 12–29 (1982).

McEachron, D. L.; Kripke, D. F.; Wyborney, V. G.: Lithium promotes entrainment of rats to long circadian light-dark cycles. Psychiat. Res. *5:* 1–9 (1981).

Naber, D.; Wirz-Justice, A.; Kafka, M. S.: Circadian rhythm in rat brain opiate receptor. Neurosci. Lett. *21:* 45–50 (1981).

Naber, D.; Wirz-Justice, A.; Kafka, M. S.: Chronic fluphenazine treatment modifies circadian rhythms of neurotransmitter receptor binding in rat brain. J. neural Transm. *55:* 277–288 (1982).

Naber, D.; Wirz-Justice, A.; Kafka, M.S.; Wehr, T.A.: Dopamine receptor binding in rat striatum: ultradian rhythm and its modification by chronic imipramine. Psychopharmacology 68: 1–5 (1980).

Papousek, M.: Chronobiologische Aspekte der Zyklothymie. Fortschr. Neurol. Psychiatr. 43: 381–440 (1975).

Pittendrigh, C.S.; Caldarola, P.C.: General homeostasis of the frequency of circadian oscillations. Proc. natn. Acad. Sci. USA 70: 2697–2701 (1973).

Pittendrigh, C.S.; Daan, S.: A functional analysis of circadian pacemakers in nocturnal rodents. I. The stability and lability of spontaneous frequency. J. comp. Physiol. 106: 223–252 (1976).

Pflug, B.; Tölle, R.: Disturbance of the 24-hour rhythm in endogenous depression and the treatment of endogenous depression by sleep deprivation. Int. Pharmacopsychiat. 6: 187–196 (1971).

Potter, W.Z.; Murphy, D.L.; Wehr, T.A.; Linnoila, M.; Goodwin, F.K.: Clorgyline: a new treatment for patients with refractory rapid cycling disorder. Archs gen. Psychiat. 39: 505–510 (1982).

Richter, C.P.: Biological clocks in medicine and psychiatry (Thomas, Springfield 1965).

Strumwasser, F.; Viele, D.P.: Lithium increases the period of the neuronal circadian oscillator. Abstr. 241.5. 10th Annu. Meet. Soc. Neurosci. (1980).

Turek, F.W.; Gwinner, E.: Role of hormones in the circadian organization of vertebrates; in Aschoff, Daan, Groos, Vertebrate circadian systems: structure and physiology, pp. 173–182 (Springer, Heidelberg 1982).

Wehr, T.A.; Goodwin, F.K.: Rapid cycling in manic-depressives induced by tricyclic antidepressants. Archs gen. Psychiat. 36: 555–559 (1979).

Wehr, T.A.; Goodwin, F.K.: Biological rhythms and psychiatry; in Arieti, Brodie, American handbook of psychiatry, vol. 7, pp. 46–74 (Basic Books, New York 1981).

Wehr, T.A.; Goodwin, F.K.; Wirz-Justice, A.; Breitmaier, J.; Craig, C.: 48-hour sleep-wake cycles in manic-depressive illness: naturalistic observations and sleep deprivation experiments. Archs gen. Psychiat. 39: 559–565 (1982a).

Wehr, T.A.; Lewy, A.J.; Wirz-Justice, A.; Craig, C.; Tamarkin, L.: Antidepressants and a circadian rhythm phase advance hypothesis of depression; in Collin, Ducharme, Barbeau, Tolis, Brain peptides and hormones, pp. 263–276 (Raven Press, New York 1982b).

Wehr, T.A.; Wirz-Justice, A.: Internal coincidence model for sleep deprivation and depression; in Koella, Sleep 1980. Proc. 5th Eur. Congr. Sleep Res., Amsterdam 1980, pp. 26–33 (Karger, Basel 1981).

Wehr, T.A.; Wirz-Justice, A.; Goodwin, F.K.; Duncan, W.; Gillin, J.C.: Phase advance of the sleep-wake cycle as an antidepressant. Science 206: 710–713 (1979).

Wever, R.: The circadian system of man: results of experiments under temporal isolation (Springer, New York 1979).

Wirz-Justice, A.; Campbell, I.C.: Antidepressant drugs can slow or dissociate circadian rhythms. Experientia 38: 1301–1309 (1982).

Wirz-Justice, A.; Kafka, M.S.; Naber, D.; Campbell, I.C.; Marangos, P.J.; Tamarkin, L.; Wehr, T.A.: Clorgyline delays the phase-position of circadian neurotransmitter receptor rhythms. Brain Res. 241: 115–122 (1982a).

Wirz-Justice, A.; Groos, G.A.; Wehr, T.A.: The neuropharmacology of circadian timekeeping in mammals; in Aschoff, Daan, Groos, Vertebrate circadian systems: structure and physiology, pp. 183–193 (Springer, Heidelberg 1982b).

Wirz-Justice A.; Kafka, M. S.; Naber, D.; Wehr, T. A.: Circadian rhythms in rat brain α- and β-adrenergic receptors are modified by chronic imipramine. Life Sci. 27: 341–347 (1980).

Wirz-Justice, A.; Tobler, I.; Kafka, M. S.; Naber, D.; Marangos, P. J.; Borbély, A. A.; Wehr, T. A.: Sleep deprivation: effects on circadian rhythms of rat brain neurotransmitter receptors. Psychiat. Res. 5: 67–76 (1981).

Wirz-Justice, A. Wehr, T. A.: Uncoupling of circadian rhythms in hamsters and man; in Sleep 1980. Proc. 5th Eur. Congr. Sleep Res., Amsterdam 1980, pp. 64–72 (Karger, Basel 1981).

Anna Wirz-Justice, PhD, Psychiatrische Universitätsklinik, Wilhelm-Klein-Strasse 27, CH-4025 Basel (Switzerland)

Adv. biol. Psychiat., vol. 11, pp. 35–47 (Karger, Basel 1983)

Tolerance to Shift Work: A Chronobiological Approach[1]

Alain Reinberg[a], *Norbert Vieux*[b], *Pierre Andlauer*[c], *Michael Smolensky*[d]

[a] ER CNRS de Chronobiologie humaine, Fondation A. de Rothschild, Paris, France; [b] Service Médical Shell Française, Petit-Couronne, France; [c] Service Médical Gilette, Annecy, France, and [d] School of Public Health, University of Texas, Health Science Center at Houston, Tex., USA

Introduction

Studies summarized in this paper were performed to provide biologically validated answers to the following questions posed by both shift workers and industrial managers, namely: (1) Why are only certain subjects able to tolerate shift work for many years? (2) Are there chronobiological criteria or indices predictive of shift-work capacity or tolerance? These questions were addressed in field studies performed between 1971 and 1981 by members of our group under specified experimental conditions using chronobiological investigative methods [*Reinberg*, 1979; *Reinberg* et al., 1981a, b]. Pertinent to this meeting and to questions 1 and 2 are the following clinical findings [*Reinberg* et al., 1981a]: an internal desynchronization (i.e., alteration of the phase relationship) of certain circadian rhythms may be associated with major affective disorders, e.g., depression [*Kripke*, 1981] as well as intolerance to shift work [*Andlauer* et al., 1979] in predisposed subjects. Despite the fact that depression and intolerance to shift work have a different pathogenesis, both exhibit a striking similarity with regard to: (1) clinical symptoms, and (2) some presumably pathological alterations of subjects' temporal structure manifested as an internal desynchronization of circadian rhythms.

[1] This work was supported by DGRST (RESACT) grant No. 79.7.1105 and Shell Française. Special thanks are due to Dr. *Daniel F. Kripke*, University of California, San Diego, and to Dr. *Alena Bicakova-Rocher*, Hôpital F. Widal, Université de Paris VII.

Chronobiological Adjustment to a 'New' Activity-Rest Schedule after a Shift

A circadian rhythm with a period, τ ($\cong 24$ h) can be characterized by specific endpoints: acrophase, $\emptyset$ (crest time, along the 24-hour scale, of the best fitting cosine function approximating all data); amplitude, A (half of the total peak-to-trough variability) and mesor, M (24-hour rhythm-adjusted mean) which approximates the arithmetic mean when data forming the time series are collected at equal time intervals [*Halberg and Reinberg*, 1967; *Halberg* et al., 1972].

A phase shift ($\Delta\psi$) of socioecological synchronizers, such as the clock hours corresponding to sleep and activity, typically is followed by an acrophase shift ($\Delta\emptyset$) which is in the same direction and magnitude as the $\Delta\psi$. Common examples of $\Delta\psi$ in human beings are provided by transmeridian flights across at least 5 time zones and shift work with $\Delta\psi \cong 8$ h involving abrupt changes from either day-work/night-sleep to night-work/day-sleep or the reverse.

Previous studies [*Halberg and Reinberg*, 1967; *Rutenfranz*, 1978; *Reinberg*, 1970; *Aschoff* et al., 1975; *Klein* et al., 1979, 1980] have shown that the span of time needed to adjust ($\Delta\emptyset \cong \Delta\psi$) from an 'old' to a 'new' schedule after a $\Delta\psi$ varies: (a) from variable to variable in the same subject; (b) with the direction of the $\Delta\psi$ ($\emptyset$ s adjust faster after a phase delay, such as in a flight from Europe to USA, than after a phase advance, such as in a flight from USA to Europe), and (c) between subjects for the span of time needed to adjust (speed of adjustment) for a given variable. The present paper concerns mainly interindividual changes of type c above.

Clinical Criteria of Intolerance to Shift Work

Only a limited (as yet not quantified) number of apparently healthy human adults can sustain shift work for an appreciable number of years [*Åkersted*, 1976; *Landier and Vieux*, 1976; *Andlauer* et al., 1977]. Some can adhere to shift work throughout their active working life (35 or more years) without medical problems or complaints. Yet, even many young workers suffer persisting fatigue, sleep disturbance and other symptoms after just a few months of shift work. But clinical symptoms of intolerance may be seen as well after one or two decades of shift work in some presumably tolerant workers when 40–50 years of age.

The clinical intolerance to shift is appreciated conventionally by considering both the existence and the intensity of a set of shift-work associated medical problems. *Sleep alterations* consisting of subjective self-ratings of poor sleep quality, difficulty of falling asleep, frequent awakening, insomnia, etc., are common complaints of intolerant shift workers. *Persisting fatigue* is another problem; the employee is often tired on awakening and not rested after sleep, weekends or vacations. This differs from physiological fatigue due to physical and/or mental effort; the latter disappears after adequate rest. *Changes in behavior* consist of unusual irritability, tantrum, malaise and inadequate performance, etc. *Digestive troubles* include various common complaints ranging from dyspepsia and epigastric pain to peptic ulcer.

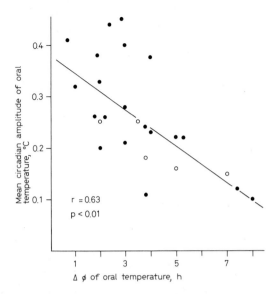

Fig. 1. Correlation between individual mean amplitude (in °C) and acrophase shift $\Delta\varnothing$ (in h) of the oral temperature circadian rhythm. $\Delta\varnothing$ corresponds to the difference of $\varnothing$ locations on the 24-hour scale between control days and the first night shift (night work from 21.00 to 05.00 or 06.00 associated with day sleep). ● = 20 shift workers, Reichstett study; ○ = 5 shift workers, Petit-Couronne study.

The symptoms of depression [*Eisenberg*, 1981] are in many ways similar to those of shift-work intolerance. However, symptoms of the latter disappear usually when the subject ceases shift work and, in addition, without the need for antidepressive drugs. Incidentally, an important indication of intolerance to shift work is the *regular use of sleeping pills* of any kind.

Chronobiological Indices of Intolerance to Shift Work

Currently, methods do not exist to predetermine whether a subject will exhibit long-term tolerance to shift work. Only by on-the-job experience is it possible to estimate one's capability. Therefore, our experimental strategy for evaluating chronobiological indices of shift-work intolerance was, and still is, to compare characteristics of biological rhythms between groups of subjects differing only by the fact they do or do not tolerate shift work. A series of studies were performed to test two major hypotheses. Since material, methods and results of these experiments were published in

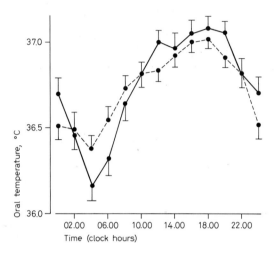

Fig. 2. Circadian changes in oral temperature rhythm of subjects tolerant and nontolerant to shift work (chronograms). Pooled data from measurements performed in subgroups of subjects —— = Tolerant to shift work; – – – = nontolerant to shift work. For each time point (every other hour) respective means ($\overline{X} \pm 1\,SE$) are plotted on a 24-hour scale.

several papers [*Reinberg* et al., 1978, 1980, 1981 a, b; *Andlauer* et al., 1979], only the major relevant findings are summarized here.

Is a Large Circadian Amplitude of Oral Temperature Associated with a
Slow Phase Shift in Circadian Rhythms of Shift Workers? [*Reinberg*
et al., 1978]

Aschoff [1978] and *Wever* [1979] in experiments conducted under conditions of temporal isolation observed the circadian amplitude of certain variables, such as oral temperature, to be a chronobiological index of one's ability to phase shift circadian rhythms. Our aim was to test the validity of *Aschoff's* [1978] hypothesis that persons with a large circadian temperature amplitude adjust more slowly than those with a small amplitude.

Figure 1 shows the negative correlation obtained between the circadian amplitude and $\Delta \phi$ for oral temperature ($r = -0.63$; $p < 0.01$) of 25 male *tolerant* (at the time of study) shift workers employed in the oil refinery industry. The larger the amplitude, the smaller the $\Delta \phi$. A negative correlation between amplitude and $\Delta \phi$ was also demonstrated for the urinary 17-OHCS ($r = -0.60$; $p < 0.01$) circadian rhythm.

Is a Large Circadian Rhythm Amplitude of Oral Temperature
Indicative of Good Clinical Tolerance to Shift Work? [Andlauer et al.,
1979; *Reinberg* et al., 1980]

This second hypothesis was proposed by *Andlauer* et al., [1977]. Inspection of the raw data of 25 shift workers lead these investigators to suspect that a large circadian amplitude oral temperature rhythm is associated with good tolerance to shift work. Four different studies were done dealing with different types of work in the steel, chemical and oil industries utilizing employees adhering to different rotation schedules (shifts every 3–4 days and every 7 days) and with groups differing in age as well as seniority involving, overall, 97 male subjects. These studies, as well as another by *Leonard* [1981] in Belgium on coal miners, confirm the fact that a large amplitude is associated with good tolerance to shift work (fig. 2).

Compatibility and Complementarity of the Tested Hypothesis: a
Tolerant Shift Worker with a Large Circadian Amplitude of
Temperature Rhythm Adjusts Slowly and/or Partially after a Shift
[*Reinberg* et al., 1980, 1981a, b]

It appears that tolerant subjects who are resistant to the effects of shift work have a large circadian amplitude of oral temperature and adjust slowly and only partially after $\Delta\psi$. Nontolerant subjects having medical complaints and revealing a certain fragility have a small circadian amplitude temperature rhythm and a rapid and frequently complete adjustment ($\Delta\phi \cong \Delta\psi$) a shift (table I).

Are These Complementary Hypotheses Valid for Variables Other than
Temperature? [Reinberg et al., 1981a, b]

Tolerant and nontolerant shift workers, oil refinery operators, in their fifties and with, respectively, 26.1 and 23.2 years seniority in shift-work positions were studied. Each self-measured at 4-hour intervals (not during sleep) 5 times/24 h their grip strength, peak expiratory flow (an index of the bronchial patency) and heart rate in addition to oral temperature. The study lasted from 24 to 28 days. Shift rotation occurred every 3–4 days (rapid rotation). The grip strength circadian amplitude was greater in shift workers with good tolerance ($14.2 \pm 1.9\%$ mean amplitude ± 1 SE) than in those with poor tolerance (7.5 ± 0.5; $p < 0.01$). A negative correlation ($r = -0.52$; $p < 0.05$) was found between the circadian amplitude of grip strength and its $\Delta\phi$. The temperature amplitude of tolerant shift workers

Table I. Circadian rhythm in oral temperature of subjects with good, adequate or poor tolerance to shift work: single cosinor summary

Group (Mean age, years)	Tolerance to shift-work (number of subjects)	Rhythm detection p	Mesor 24-hour-rhythm-adjusted mean ± 1 SE (°C)	Amplitude °C (95 % confidence limit)	Acrophase ∅ in h and min, ∅ reference: midnight = 00.00 95 % confidence limit
I 25.3	good (6)	<0.005	36.53 ± 0.08	0.37 (0.29–0.45)	15.49 (14.38 to 17.00)
II 50.0	good (10)	<0.005	36.51 ± 0.07	0.35 (0.30–0.40)	15.34 (15.21 to 16.27)
III 50.2	adeq. (6)	<0.005	36.53 ± 0.11	0.30 (0.24–0.36)	16.57 (15.41 to 19.05)
IV 47.4	poor (7)	<0.005	36.52 ± 0.12	0.23 (0.17–0.29)	17.11 (16.07 to 18.14)

All subjects were shift workers at the same oil refinery. Groups differed mainly by a good (e. g., group II) versus a poor (group IV) tolerance to shift work as well as by a large (group II) versus a small (group IV) amplitude. Group II (good tolerance) involved 10 senior operators (no history of shift-work difficulty; mean age = 50 years, range 44–57 years; and mean shift-work duration = 25.1 years, range 15–32 years). Group IV involved 7 senior operators (who were to be discharged from shift work due to nontolerance; mean age = 47.4 years, range 30–56 years; mean shift-work duration = 22.9 years, range 9–29).

Notes: In any group, amplitude differs from zero with $p < 0.005$; mesor: no difference between groups; amplitude (½ of total variability). large in groups I and II (good tolerance); small in group IV (poor tolerance to shift-work); acrophase ∅ (crest time): no difference between groups.

was greater ($0.31 \pm 0.06°C$) than that of nontolerant shift workers ($0.15 \pm 0.03°C$; $p < 0.04$). There was a negative correlation ($r = -0.67$; $p < 0.01$) between the circadian amplitude and the $\Delta \emptyset$ resulting from shift work. Thus, the circadian amplitudes of both temperature and grip strength exhibited a similar relationship to shift-work tolerance as well as $\Delta \emptyset$s.

This was not the case for the circadian rhythms of both heart rate and PEF; differences in the amplitudes between tolerant and nontolerant groups were not statistically significant. Although the $\Delta \emptyset$ of the PEF rhythm was greater for subjects with poor (4.31 ± 0.72 h) than for good tolerance (2.48 ± 0.29 h; $p < 0.05$), there was no correlation between the amplitudes and $\Delta \emptyset$s of PEF ($r = -0.13$) and for that matter for heart rate ($r = -0.10$). Apparently, the amplitude of variables such as heart rate and PEF are more influenced by external factors than are body temperature and grip strength [*Reinberg* et al., 1979; *Reinberg* et al., 1981a, b].

Table II. Oral temperature (cosinor summary)

Subject's age years	Rhythm detection p	Mesor 24-hour adjusted mean ± 1 SE	Amplitude 95 % confidence limit	Acrophase ϕ in h and min, ϕ reference: midnight 95 % confidence limit
53	<0.005	36.33 ± 0.006	0.22 (0.18–0.25)	14.49 (13.55 to 15.40)
55	<0.005	36.54 ± 0.003	0.32 (0.28–0.35)	15.52 (15.29 to 16.15)
55	<0.05	36.59 ± 0.002	0.03 (0.00–0.06)	12.47 (08.17 to 17.17)
50	<0.005	36.54 ± 0.005	0.18 (0.14–0.22)	17.03 (16.18 to 17.55)
32	<0.005	36.48 ± 0.015	0.48 (0.41–0.56)	17.12 (16.40 to 17.48)
GT	<0.002	36.46 ± 0.002	0.23 (0.20–0.26)	17.39 (17.09 to 18.10)

5 senior operators discharged from shift work for 1.5–4 years after becoming nontolerant after 11–23 years of shift work. Subject's synchronization: light-on at 06.30 ± 1 h; light-off at 23.00 ± 1 h.
Notes: mesor and amplitude given in °C. Data of another group of senior operators with good tolerance (GT) to shift work are taken as reference.

Oral Temperature Circadian Rhythm Parameters of Former Shift Workers with Poor Tolerance

5 senior operators between 32 and 55 years of age had been working shifts for between 11 and 23 years before becoming nontolerant. Between 1½ and 4 years prior to their study, a diurnal work schedule was resumed resulting in the remedy of their former shift-work-related medical problems. Self-rated characteristics of sleep during 25 nights showed a high percentage rated as 'good' or 'excellent', a low percentage of fatigue upon awaking and a good continuity of sleep, i.e., low frequency of spontaneous awakeness. In addition, 4 of the 5 senior operators had a large circadian temperature amplitude (table II). Only one had a circadian amplitude lower than either the amplitudes of the other 4 subjects or the mean amplitude of a group of tolerant shift workers, which served as a control group. This finding is in favor of the hypothesis that the clinical symptoms of poor tolerance to shift work as well as the alteration in amplitude observed in some shift workers are reversible.

Circadian Time Structure Alterations in Nontolerant Shift Workers, Depressive Patients and Apparently Healthy Subjects

According to *Aschoff* et al. [1975], *Aschoff* [1978] and *Wever* [1979], the circadian rhythms of body temperature and the sleep-wake cycle depend on two different biological oscillators. When a subject's circadian rhythms are entrained by regular (non-shifting) synchronizers or external zeitgebers (with a period, $\tau \cong 24$ h), these two (at least) oscillators apparently run more or less synchronously. However, when synchronizers are manipulated, such as during temporal isolation without time cue and clue or shift work, they may run more or less independently with different periods leading to an internal desynchronization of rhythms and an alteration of the subject's temporal organization. Emphasis must be given to the fact that interindividual differences can be demonstrated in terms of both synchronization and desynchronization of circadian rhythms as well as alteration of the temporal structure.

Tolerant Shift Workers

It is likely that a subject with good shift-work tolerance for many years (e. g., at the age of 44–57 years after 15–32 years of shift work) has a large circadian amplitude of both body temperature and grip strength and adjusts slowly after a $\Delta\psi$. In other terms, it seems that such a subject has a 'strong' temporal organization with reference to the fact that at least these rhythms are little affected for many years by repeated $\Delta\phi$ s.

Nontolerant Shift Workers

Both small amplitudes and large $\Delta\phi$ s of circadian temperature and grip strength rhythms were observed in subjects who abruptly (within 3–6 months) developed symptoms of intolerance after many years of shift work. Detection of a weak temporal structure, defined by low amplitudes and rapid $\Delta\phi$ s after $\Delta\psi$ s, in these subjects is consistent with a heightened susceptibility to internal desynchronization among certain circadian rhythms and/or systems.

Depression

Many studies have been devoted to a presumable relationship between an internal desynchronization and affective illnesses [*Halberg*, 1967; *Kripke* et al., 1978; *Kripke*, 1981; *Wehr* et al., 1979, 1980]. The first hypothesis proposed by *Halberg* [1967] is that manic-depressive cycles might result from a beat phenomenon between desynchronized rhythms. *Kripke* et al. [1978] showed in some patients that the period of a set of rhythms was shorter than 24 h (e. g., $\tau \cong 21.8$ h) and that depression occurred as the body temperature phase advanced. *Wehr* et al. [1980] found in comparison to healthy controls that several circadian rhythmic variables, in addition to body temperature, exhibited statistically significant phase advances in both depressed and manic patients. A variety of evidence suggests a relationship between internal desynchronization, involving alterations of the circadian rhythm period and/ or acrophase, and affective illnesses. However, to be more specific in attempting to correlate a given affective syndrome to a given circadian rhythm disorder sufficient data are lacking.

Apparently Healthy Subjects

An internal desynchronization of certain circadian rhythms, such as oral temperature and systolic blood pressure, has been demonstrated by

Bickova-Rocher et al. [1981] in 6 of 12 apparently healthy subjects synchronized with diurnal activity and nocturnal rest. Subjects with rhythm alterations had low a circadian amplitude and an unstable ϕ location without symptoms of a physiologic dysfunction, including poor or bad sleep. This means that an internal desynchronization may occur without $\Delta\psi$ and does not lead, by itself, to symptoms of depression. Other factors, in addition to rhythm alterations, must be considered to explain why only certain subjects suffer from depression or intolerance to shift work. We fully agree with *Kripke* et al. [1981] who stated:

'It would appear that internal desynchronization of rhythms does not always or usually cause serious affective disturbances, but internal desynchronization may be associated with extremely serious depression among occasional subjects. ... It is conceivable that internal desynchronization of rhythms produces major affective disorders only among those subjects who are genetically, biologically, and perhaps also psychologically predisposed.'

Circumstances and Conditions of the Internal Desynchronization in Depression and Intolerance to Shift Work

Depression

Internal desynchronization appears to be related mainly to endogenous factors. The period of circadian oscillators is under genetic control. Therefore, a genetic predisposition to depression may depend upon genetic changes in the circadian oscillator or its phasing. However, environmental factors, including synchronizer manipulation, may play a role in certain conditions and certain subjects.

Intolerance to Shift Work

Internal desynchronization, i. e., alteration in the phase relationship of biological rhythms, is predominantly related to manipulation of the subject's synchronizer as is the case shift work. Yet, only certain (prone?) employes develop intolerance. This raises the question of a predisposition (occurring at a given age?) to suffer the symptoms of depression as well as exhibiting rhythms with small amplitudes and large $\Delta\phi$s. Studying the pathological consequences of shift work in retired workers, *Michel-Briand* et al. [1981] reported there were more cases of depression and affective illness in retired shift workers than in retired day workers in whom cardiovascular and locomotor problems were more predominant. It could well be that in predisposed subjects an internal desynchronization is associated with symptoms which are common to both depression and shift-work intolerance. This is not to imply we are dealing with either two different diseases or two clinical forms of the same disease.

The studies of *Yunis* et al. [1973, 1974] are pertinent to considering genetic predispositions to disease. Circadian amplitudes and ϕs of the rectal temperature rhythm in mice of different strains (mainly CBA and NZB) were quantified in relation to both $\Delta\psi$s (simulating shift work) and to aging. The speed of adjustment, the circadian rhythm amplitude as well as respective changes in each with aging are presumably of genetic origin.

Effective Treatments May Contribute to the Control of Internal Desynchronization

Depression

Lithium [*Engelmann,* 1973; *Kripke* et al., 1978; *Johnsson* et al., 1979] and to a certain extent other antidepressant drugs [*Halberg,* 1963; *Wirz-Justice* et al., 1980a, b] used to control depression and manic-depressive illness have been shown to act on the period of certain circadian rhythms. Manipulation of synchronizers, e. g., a 6-hour phase advance of the sleep/wake cycle, appears to be an effective treatment of chronic depression according to *Wehr* et al. [1979].

Intolerant Shift Workers

As a rule, nontolerant shift workers develop a kind of addiction to sleeping pills (barbiturates, tranquilizers, benzodiazepin derivatives, antihistamines, etc.). Emphasis must be given to the fact that biomedical problems of intolerance to shift work cannot be solved by medications. Return to a regular synchronization, with duirnal activity and nocturnal rest within 6 months after the commencement of symptoms, usually alleviates both the clinical symptoms and circadian rhythm alterations of shift-work intolerance. However, the medical decision to discharge a nontolerant subject from shift work must be taken early.

Conclusions

1. It could be of interest to study the circadian rhythm amplitude in depressive patients as well as to research criteria for primary depression and family histories of affective disorders in apparently healthy shift workers.

2. The overall amplitude of the circadian rhythm in body temperature and grip strength is likely to be a good candidate, among others yet to be found, as a chronobiological index of the long-term ability to tolerate shift work.

3. If persisting tolerance to shift work throughout one's lifetime is associated with a large circadian amplitude and slow adjustment of both temperature and grip strength rhythms, a type of shift schedule not allowing the worker adjustment to a 'new' synchronization has to be preferred. Therefore, a rapid rotation, with shifts every 2–3 days, seems to be a better choice than the conventional weekly rotation. Such a rapid rotation may help to minimize the potential risk of an internal desynchronization.

Summary

Clinical criteria of intolerance to shift work (sleep disturbances, persisting fatigue, behavioral and gastrointestinal troubles) were taken into consideration in the research of chronobiological indices predictive of tolerance to shift work. Employees nontolerant to shift work have a relatively small circadian amplitude of body temperature and adjust rather quickly with a rapid acrophase shift in both the body temperature and grip strength rhythms following alteration in the rest/activity schedule. Rhythms of small amplitude, implying a weak temporal organization of biological functions, presumably are predisposing to internal desynchronization. Similarities and differences between depression and intolerance to shift work are discussed with regard to clinical symptoms, type of rhythm alterations, origin of the internal desynchronization, treatment and prevention.

References

Åkerstedt, T.: Interindividual differences in adjustment to shift-work. Proc. 6th Int. Congr. Ergonomics, pp.510–514 (Human Factor Society, Santa Monica 1976).

Andlauer, P.; Carpentier, J.; Cazamian, P.: Ergonomie du travail de nuit et des horaires alternants. Education permanente. Université de Paris I (Editions Cujas, Paris 1977).

Andlauer, P.; Reinberg, A.; Fourré, L.; Battle, W.; Duverneuil, G.: Amplitude of the oral temperature circadian rhythm and the tolerance to shift-work. J. physiol., Paris 75: 507–512 (1979).

Aschoff, J.: Features of circadian rhythms relevant for the design of shift schedules. Ergonomics 39: 739–754 (1978).

Aschoff, J.; Hoffmann, K.; Pohl, H.; Wever, R.: Reentrainment of circadian rhythms after phase-shifts of the Zeitgeber. Chronobiologia 2: 23–78 (1975).

Bicakova-Rocher, A.; Gorceix, A.; Reinberg, A.: Possible circadian rhythm alterations in certain healthy human adults before and during the administration of a pseudo-drug; in Reinberg, Vieux, Andlauer, Night and shift-work studies: biological and social aspects, pp.297–310 (Pergamon Press, Oxford 1981).

Eisenberg, L.: La dépression nerveuse. Recherche 12: 160–172 (1981).

Engelmann, W.: A slowing down of circadian rhythms by lithium ions. Z. Naturf. 28c: 733–736 (1973).

Halberg, F.: Circadian rhythms in experimental medicine. Proc. R. Soc. Med. *56:* 253–256 (1963).

Halberg, F.: Physiologic considerations underlying rhythmometry, with special reference to emotional illness; in de Ajuriaguerra, Symposium Bel-Air III, Cycle biologiques et psychiatrie, pp. 73–126 (Masson, Paris 1967).

Halberg, F.; Johnsson, E. A.; Nelson, W.; Runge, W.; Sothern, R.: Autorhythmometry procedures for physiologic self-measurements and their analysis. Physiol. Teacher *1:* 1–11 (1972).

Halberg, F.; Reinberg, A.: Rythmes circadiens et rythmes de basses fréquences en physiologie humaine. J. Physiol., Paris *59:* 117–200 (1967).

Johnsson, A.; Pflug, B.; Engelmann, W.; Klemke, W.: Effect of lithium carbonate on circadian periodicity in humans. Pharmakopsychiatr. Neuro-Psychopharmakol. *12:* 423–425 (1979).

Klein, K. E.; Wegmann, H. M.: Circadian rhythms of human performance and resistance: operational aspects; in Nicholson, Sleep wakefulness and circadian rhythms. AGARD lecture series, No. 105, pp. 2-1–2-17 (AGARD NATO, Neuilly sur Seine 1979).

Klein, K. E.; Wegmann, H. M.: Significance of circadian rhythms in aerospace operations. AGARDograph No. 247, p. 60 (AGARD NATO, Neuilly sur Seine 1980).

Kripke, D. F.: Phase advance theories for affective illnesses; in Goodwin, Wehr, Circadian rhythms in psychiatry: basic and clinical studies (Boxwood Press, California, in press 1981).

Kripke, D. F.; Mullaney, D. J.; Atkinson, M.; Wolf, S.: Circadian rhythm disorders in manic-depressives. Biol. Psychiat. *13:* 335–351 (1978).

Landier, H.; Vieux, N.: Le travail posté en question (Edition du Cerf, Paris 1976).

Leonard, R.: Amplitude of the temperature circadian rhythm and tolerance to shift-work; in Reinberg, Vieux, Andlauer, Night and shift-work studies: biological and social aspects, pp. 323–329 (Pergamon Press, Oxford 1981).

Michel-Briand, C.; Chopard, J. L.; Guiot, A.; Paulmeier, M.; Struder, G.: The pathological consequences of shift-work in retired workers; in Reinberg, Vieux, Andlauer, Night and shift-work studies: biological and social aspects, pp. 399–407 (Pergamon Press, Oxford 1981).

Reinberg, A.: Evaluation of circadian dyschronism during transmeridian flights. Studium gen. *23:* 1159–1168 (1970).

Reinberg, A.: Chronobiological field studies of oil refinery shift workers. Chronobiologia *6:* suppl. 1, p. 119 (1979).

Reinberg, A.; Andlauer, P.; Guillet, P.; Nicolai, A.: Oral temperature, circadian rhythm amplitude, ageing and tolerance to shift-work. Ergonomics *23:* 55–64 (1980).

Reinberg, A.; Smolensky, M.; Vieux, N.; Andlauer, P.: Chronobiological field studies of shift-workers: indices of individual tolerance: feeding patterns, in Czeisler, Moore-Ede, Weitzman, Circadian clocks in man: time keeping in health and disease (in press, 1981a).

Reinberg, A.; Vieux, N.; Andlauer, P.; Guillet, P.; Nicolai, A.: Tolerance of shift-work, amplitude of circadian rhythms and aging; in Reinberg, Vieux, Andlauer, Night and shift-work studies: biological and social aspects, pp. 341–354 (Pergamon Press, Oxford 1981b).

Reinberg, A.; Vieux, N.; Chaumont, A. J.; Laporte, A.; Smolensky, M.; Nicolai, A.; Abulker, C.; Dupont, J.: Aims and conditions of shift-work studies. Chronobiologia *6:* suppl. 1, pp. 7–26 (1979).

Reinberg, A.; Vieux, N.; Ghata, J.; Chaumont, A.J.; Laporte, A.: Is the rhythm amplitude related to the ability to phase-shift circadian rhythms of shift-workers? J. Physiol., Paris 74: 405–409 (1978).

Rutenfranz, J.: Schichtarbeit und biologische Rhythmik. Arzneimittel-Forsch. 28: 1867–1872 (1978).

Wehr, T.A.; Muscetolla, G.; Goodwin, F.K.: Urinary 3-methoxy-4-hydroxyphenylglycol circadian rhythms. Archs gen. Psychiat. 37: 257–263 (1980).

Wehr, T.A.; Wirz-Justice, A.; Goodwin, F.K.; Duncan, W.; Gillin, J.C.: Phase advance of the circadian sleep-wake cycle as an antidepressant. Science 206: 710–713 (1979).

Wever, R.A.: The circadian system of man. Results of experiments under temporal isolation (Springer, New York 1979).

Wirz-Justice, A.; Kafka, M.S.; Naber, D.; Wehr, T.A.: Circadian rhythms in rat brain alpha- and beta-adrenergic receptors are modified by chronic imipramine. Life Sci. 27: 341–347 (1980a).

Wirz-Justice, A.; Wehr, T.A.; Goodwin, F.K.; Kafka, M.S.; Naber, D.; Marangos, P.J.; Campbell, I.C.: Antidepressant drugs slow circadian rhythms in behaviour and brain neurotransmitter receptors. Psychopharmacol. Bull. 16: 45–47 (1980b).

Yunis, E.J.; Halberg, F.; McMullen, A.; Ruitman, B.; Fernandes, G.: Model studies of aging, genetic and stable versus changing living routine simulated by lighting regimen manipulation on the mouse. Int. J. Chronobiol. 1: 368–369 (1973).

Yunis, E.J.; Fernandes, G.; Nelson, W.; Halberg, F.: Circadian temperature rhythms and aging in rodents; in Scheving, Halberg, Pauly, Chronobiology, pp.358–363 (Igaku Shoin, Tokyo 1974).

Addendum

Since the presentation of this paper a desynchronization of the oral temperature circadian rhythm of young subjects with poor tolerance for night work was demonstrated. 11 subjects with good tolerance had (with one exception) the prominent circadian period τ equal to 24 h. By contrast subjects with poor tolerance had a τ value ranging from 24.9 to 25.7 h associated with a relatively small rhythm amplitude.

Reinberg, A.; Andlauer, P.; Teinturier, P.; De Prins, J.; Malbecq, W.; Dupont, J.: C.r. hebd. Séanc. Acad. Sci, Paris (in press).

A. Reinberg, MD, ER CNRS de Chronobiologie humaine, Fondation A. de Rothschild, 29, rue Manin, F-75940 Paris Cedex 19 (France)

Adv. biol. Psychiat., vol. 11, pp. 48–59 (Karger, Basel 1983)

Endocrine Rhythms in a Nonhuman Primate, the Rhesus Monkey[1]

Hans-Jürgen Quabbe, Michael Gregor, Christine Bumke-Vogt, Ingrid Witt, Daniel Giannella-Neto

Section of Endocrinology, Department of Internal Medicine, Klinikum Steglitz, Freie Universität, Berlin, FRG

Introduction

The central nervous system (CNS) has intrinsic rhythmogenic properties. These are subject to modulation by external cues (e. g. light). On the other hand, the CNS transmits rhythmic information to the body via peripheral nervous pathways and the endocrine system. Although the latter is usually thought to act by hypothalamic regulation of pituitary hormone secretion, a direct influence of the CNS on peripheral glands via autonomic nerves is also possible. In reverse, circulating hormones (e. g. glucocorticosteroids) can modulate CNS rhythms.

In psychosomatic and psychiatric disorders, the concomitant disturbances of endocrine rhythms are often regarded as mere epiphenomena of the underlying CNS disease process. However, the interdependence of central and peripheral rhythms makes it likely that alterations in hormonal feedback may soon become part of the overall pathology.

The elucidation of the mechanisms by which CNS and endocrine rhythms are coupled to each other necessitates an animal model. In view of the involvement of higher CNS structures and because of the interest of such studies for the understanding of psychosomatic processes, the experimental animals should be as close to man as possible.

[1] Original work of the author was supported by Deutsche Forschungsgemeinschaft, SPP Neuroendokrinologie. Technical assistance was given by Ms. *M. Rösick* and Ms. *B. Hennig.* Secretarial help was provided by Ms. *J. Weirowski.*

We have studied the 24-hour secretory pattern of growth hormone (GH), prolactin (PRL), thyrotropin (TSH), thyroxine (T4) and cortisol in the male rhesus monkey with a special interest in a possible relation to the sleep/wake cycle, the daytime rest/activity cycle and the night-time sleep stage cycle. Our results provide evidence for a difference between man and monkey in the pattern of some of these hormones. They suggest a link between the secretion of PRL – but not GH – and sleep in the rhesus monkey. Furthermore, each of the hormones reacts in a different way to environmental stimuli and/or changes in sleep and waking rhythms.

Methods

12 adolescent or adult male rhesus monkeys were adapted to chronic chair living. They lived under conditions of constant temperature and humidity with a 14/10 h (06.00–20.00–06.00 h) light/dark cycle. Water and pelleted food were available ad libitum with additional feeding of fruit and vegetables at 08.30 and 16.00 h. Females or infant animals were not in the colony. The monkeys were operatively prepared for remote blood sampling from the adjacent room and for electroencephalogram (EEG), electrooculogram (EOG) and electromyogram (EMG) recording as described elsewhere [1]. During experiments, the animals were observed by closed circuit television during day and night. They always remained within their established social relations.

Blood sampling was performed every 15 min for 24 h (96 h in 4 animals) or shorter periods of time. During daytime, behavior was rated as active, quiet or napping at 5-min intervals. During the night, EEG/EOG/EMG were continuously recorded. 5 h nap (08.00–13.00 h) and 5 h sleep (20.00–01.00 h) deprivation was done by the presence of a familiar person in the animal quarters, while slow wave sleep (SWS) and rapid eye movement (REM) sleep deprivation (20.00–06.00 h) was done by the activation of a noise generator whenever the forbidden sleep stage appeared on the EEG record. Evidence for the absence of acute or chronic stress during these living conditions and during the experiments as well as further details of the methods used in these studies have been presented elsewhere [2].

Statistical Analysis

The hormonal, behavioral and EEG time series from sampling during undisturbed conditions were subjected to power spectral analysis [3] in order to detect circadian or ultradian rhythms. Cross-correlation analysis [3] between the different hormonal time series and between hormonal and behavioral/EEG time series was performed in two ways. First, cross-correlation was calculated for single pairs of time series (e.g. GH vs. PRL from any one experiment) in order to detect common periodicities. Second, correlation coefficients were calculated across groups of paired time series for short time lags (usually +60 to −60 min) in order to detect a correlation in the absence of a common periodicity. Criteria for significance and further details of the statistical analysis have been described elsewhere [1].

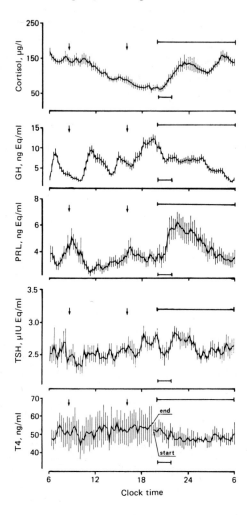

Fig1. 24-hour pattern of 5 different rhesus monkey hormones. The curves represent means (± SEM) obtained from 24-hour, daytime and night-time profiles. Vertical arrows indicate feeding of fruit and vegetables. Horizontal lines above the curves indicate time lights-off (20.00–06.00 h). Horizontal lines below the curves indicate range of sleep onset times in the respective groups of animals. The number of daytime and night-time profiles (including the respective parts of the 24-hour profiles) from which the mean concentrations have been obtained were as follows: cortisol = 45/45; GH = 45/45; PRL = 28/24; TSH = 24/22; T4 = 4/4.

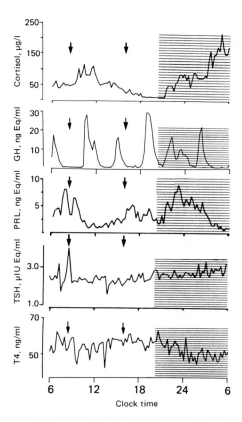

Fig. 2. Characteristic single 24-hour profiles of 5 different rhesus monkey hormones. Each profile was obtained on a different day. Vertical arrows indicate feeding of fruit and vegetables (08.30 and 16.00 h). Shaded area indicates the time the lights were off.

Results

24-Hour Pattern of Hormones

Each of the hormones which we have studied has a distinct 24-hour pattern different from the other ones. Only those of TSH and T4 are similar to each other (fig. 1, 2).

The 24-hour plasma cortisol pattern shows a 24-hour variation which is quite similar to that of man. Cortisol is high in the morning hours. It then decreases towards an evening minimum and rises again during the night. In individual curves, a period of apparent secretory arrest was sometimes present during the evening (example in fig. 2).

The 24-hour curve of mean GH concentrations shows an alternation of peaks and troughs which is more pronounced during the day and tapers off during the night. GH increases sharply at the onset of the light period (06.00 h). However, preliminary observations suggest that the sleep/wake transition rather than the dark/light transition is the synchronizer of this matutinal GH peak [*Quabbe* et al., unpubl.]. Further peaks then occur at approximately 4-hour intervals, but the troughs between the peaks become progressively more shallow due to loss of synchronization between the animals. In individual profiles, however, distinct secretory episodes continue to occur throughout the night (example in fig. 2). The highest mean concentration is reached at the end of the lights-on period, and GH begins to decrease just before sleep onset. This pattern is different from that in man in whom daytime GH secretory episodes occur less often, and a major increase usually takes place after sleep onset in relationship to SWS [4].

In the PRL curve, there are two elevations during daytime, one in the morning and a smaller one in the afternoon, which coincide with the additional feeding of fruit and vegetables. Whether this is a mere temporal coincidence or not remains to be investigated, although, in man, there is evidence that feeding does indeed have an influence on the daytime PRL pattern [5]. The most characteristic aspect of the 24-hour PRL pattern is a nocturnal elevation which begins with a steep increase of the mean 24-hour curve early in the night followed by a progressive decline thereafter until low morning values are attained. Although the early-night increase occurs within the range of sleep onset times of the animals in the curve of mean values, such a relationship was not regularly seen in individual profiles. In contrast to man [6], the highest PRL concentrations are attained early during the night and not towards the morning hours.

In contrast to these three hormones (cortisol, GH, PRL), TSH and T4 do not show any clear pattern of a nyctohemeral difference or a circadian rhythm. The TSH elevations in the late evening and during the early night with a trough in between (fig. 1) are due to the influence of a few profiles only and are not characteristic of most individual curves (example in fig. 2). In man, most investigations have shown higher nocturnal than daytime TSH concentrations [7]. Whether the lack of such a nyctohemeral difference in our animals is due to their artificial living conditions (constant temperature and humidity, restricted physical mobility) or whether it constitutes a real species difference, remains to be determined.

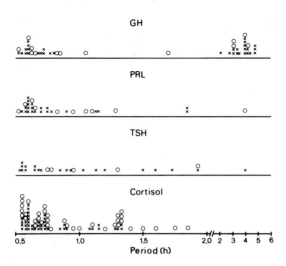

Fig. 3. Power-spectral maxima of hormonal time series. Each entry represents a power-spectral maximum from a single profile. Crosses indicate maxima with an increase of at least 50 % over a prior minimum. Open circles indicate maxima with an increase of 20–50 % over the preceding minimum.

Ultradian Periodicities

Superimposed on the larger variations during the 24-hour day, there was a high-frequency fluctuation of the plasma concentration of cortisol, PRL, TSH and T4. Only relatively few GH profiles showed a high-frequency fluctuation, although in most curves there were rudimentary GH peaks between the larger secretory episodes (example in fig. 2). Power-spectral analysis was therefore performed on the hormonal data (GH, PRL, TSH, cortisol) from undisturbed conditions (blood sampling, TV observation, EEG recording, but no disturbance of behavior) in order to detect ultradian periodicities. The results (fig. 3) indicate that all four hormones show a clustering of power-spectral maxima at periods of approximately 30–50 min and cortisol in addition at 80 min. GH is the only hormone with a predominant periodicity between 3 and 6 h. Although these power-spectral maxima are concentrated at certain periodicities, mathematically none of them proved to be significant, which points to a low expression of the underlying rhythmicity.

Table I. Cross-correlation analysis between single pairs of hormones[1]

	PRL	TSH	Cortisol
GH, all [day / night] all[2]	9 [8/27 / 1/24] 51	not calculated	23 [12/44 / 11/45] 89
PRL, all [day / night] all	–	1 [1/22 / 0/18] 40	2 [0/26 / 2/24] 50
TSH, all [day / night] all	–	–	2 [1/24 / 1/21] 45

[1] Cross-correlation was calculated separately for daytime and night-time profiles including the respective parts of the complete 24-hour profiles.
[2] Numbers of significantly correlated pairs and total number of pairs, respectively. Numbers outside the brackets indicate respective sums of the numbers for daytime and night-time pairs.

Relation of Hormones to Each Other

In order to detect possible interrelationships, cross-correlation analysis was performed between the different hormonal time series of each experiment. There was no overall common periodicity between any pair of hormones. However, in pairs from single experiments, GH and PRL were significantly correlated in 8/27 daytime profiles and GH and cortisol in 23/89 daytime and night-time profiles (table I), indicating a common periodicity of the respective hormones in these time series. The results of correlation analysis for short time lags across groups of paired time series (for which periodicity is not a prerequisite) indicate a negative correlation between PRL and GH and a positive correlation between PRL and cortisol, but only for the respective daytime profiles (table II). Apparently, a common periodicity or a nonperiodic synchronization of the episodic pattern of two or more hormones can take place under certain circumstances. The factors which determine whether synchronization occurs or not remain to be determined.

Relation to Daytime Rest/Activity Stages, to the Sleep/Wake Cycle and to Night-Time Sleep Stages

A possible relation between the hormonal pattern and daytime rest/activity stages or night-time sleep stages was first studied by cross-

Table II. Correlation analysis across groups of paired hormonal time series for short lags[1]

	PRL	TSH	Cortisol
GH	<0.01 negative[2] (daytime only)	not calculated	NS
PRL	–	NS	<0.01 positive[2] (daytime only)
TSH	–	–	NS

[1] Daytime and night-time hormonal time series (including the respective parts of the 24-hour time series) were analyzed separately. Calculation was done for time lags −60 to +60 min. NS = Absence of a significant correlation.

[2] Indicates direction of correlation.

Table III. Correlation analysis across groups of paired time series for short lags: hormones vs. daytime arousal and night-time sleep stages[1]

	GH	PRL	TSH	Cortisol
Arousal[2]	NS	<0.01 (positive)[3]		
Awake[2]	<0.01 (positive)[3]	NS	not calculated[4]	
SWS[2]	NS	NS		
REM[2]	NS	<0.1/>0.05 (negative)[3]		

NS = Absence of a significant correlation.

[1] Correlations were calculated for time lags −60 to +60 min.

[2] Daytime arousal, nocturnal stage wake and sleep stages SWS and REM, respectively.

[3] Indicates direction of correlation.

[4] Analysis across groups of paired time series was not done for TSH and cortisol, since cross-correlation for single paired time series indicated no clustering of significant cross-correlation coefficients at short time lags for these hormones.

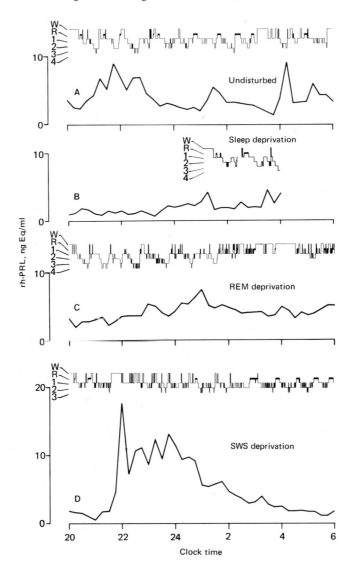

Fig. 4. Single nocturnal PRL profiles from one monkey during undisturbed conditions, 5 h sleep, REM sleep and SWS deprivation, respectively. Sleep stage profile and hormonal profile are shown for each experiment. Note sleep onset PRL increase during undisturbed conditions, its absence during total sleep deprivation and delayed rise during REM deprivation. Total sleep deprivation was done from 20.00 to 01.00 h, while REM deprivation and SWS deprivation were done from 20.00 to 06.00 h. W, R, 1, 2, 3, 4 indicate stages awake, REM sleep and non-REM sleep stages 1, 2, 3 and 4, respectively.

correlation analysis of the hormonal and the behavioral/EEG time series which were obtained during undisturbed conditions. No common periodicity was found between any of the hormones and the behavioral/EEG profiles, since all cross-correlations of single pairs of these time series were nonsignificant. However, the results of correlation analysis for short time lags across groups of paired time series indicate a positive correlation of GH to night-time awakenings and of PRL to daytime arousal. A trend for PRL to be negatively correlated with sleep stage REM failed to reach significance (table III). The positive correlation of GH to night-time awakenings may indicate a general stimulatory effect of sleep/wake transitions on GH secretion in accordance with our preliminary evidence that the matutinal GH synchronization is probably related to the sleep/wake transition. The positive relation of PRL to daytime arousal and the absence of such a relation for cortisol suggest that PRL may be a better indicator of arousal than cortisol, at least in the rhesus monkey.

Another attempt to uncover a relation of the hormonal patterns to daytime arousal, to the sleep/wake cycle and to the sleep stage cycle was made by nap, sleep and sleep stage deprivation experiments. An effect of these procedures on hormone secretion was apparent for PRL and GH. During nap deprivation, the morning peak of PRL was absent. However, this is probably nonspecific since the nap incidence was very low at this time of the morning during undisturbed conditions. During 5 h sleep deprivation, the nocturnal PRL increase did not occur and during REM deprivation it was delayed. During SWS deprivation, PRL was secreted erratically either in large bursts or during sustained periods of time, resulting in a significant increase of the mean PRL concentration, possibly as a nonspecific stress effect. An example of the PRL changes in one animal is given in figure 4. The pattern of TSH and of cortisol was essentially unchanged during all deprivation procedures, except for a cortisol increase following but not during sleep deprivation, the mechanism of which is at present unclear. Even noise levels up to 100 dB during SWS and REM deprivation did not induce an increase of the cortisol concentration.

Comment

Our studies have revealed similarities and dissimilarities of the 24-hour plasma hormone pattern between man and a nonhuman primate, the rhesus monkey. The most striking difference is an absent sleep dependence of GH

Table IV. Difference in hormone response to deprivation procedures

	Quality of deprivation procedure			
	nonstressful		potentially stressful	
	nap deprivation	sleep deprivation	SWS deprivation	REM deprivation
GH	→	↑	↑	↑
PRL	↓	↓	↑	↗
TSH	→	→	→	→
Cortisol	→	↑	→	→
		(post-deprivation)		

Symbols indicate direction of change: → = no change; ↑ = increase; ↓ = decrease; ↗ = delay of increase.
Nonstressful deprivation = Presence of a familiar person in the animal quarters who arouses the animal's attention whenever necessary by walking, speaking to the animal, etc.; potentially stressful deprivation = activation of noise generator (output up to 100 dB) whenever the forbidden sleep stage occurs in the EEG.

secretion in the monkey, while this is an important determinator of the GH pattern in man [4]. On the other hand, sleep seems to be a prerequisite for the nocturnal PRL increase in both man [6] and monkey. For TSH, a nyctohemeral difference similar to that in man [7] was not found. The cortisol pattern of man and the monkey closely resemble each other.

The analysis of our results also indicates that the episodic secretion of each hormone as well as their relation to each other respond in different and probably very complex ways to a change in the environmental conditions and/or the disruption of endogenous rhythms (arousal/napping; sleep/wake; sleep stages) (table IV). PRL and GH are more labile, while TSH and cortisol are quite insensitive. The mechanisms which determine the different patterns and responses as well as those which regulate synchronization and desynchronization of episodic hormone secretion remain largely to be determined. Different secretory patterns of some hormones in monkey and man may reflect the changing importance of certain environmental factors (light/dark cycle, presence of predators, etc.) during the evolution from nonhuman to the human primate species. Despite these differences, the rhesus monkey seems to be a valuable model for the study of endocrine rhythms and their modulation by environmental factors.

Summary

The 24-hour pattern of plasma growth hormone (GH), prolactin (PRL), thyrotropin (TSH), thyroxine (T4) and cortisol in the male rhesus monkey and their relation to the daytime rest/activity, the sleep/wake and the sleep stage cycles are described. The GH pattern differs from that in man by more frequent secretory episodes and the absence of a link to sleep. On the other hand, evidence is discussed for an influence of sleep on the pattern of PRL similar to that in man. No nyctohemeral difference was found for the TSH concentration. In contrast to GH and PRL, TSH and cortisol are largely insensitive to changes in daytime arousal, sleep or sleep stages.

References

1   Quabbe, H.-J.; Gregor, M.; Bumke-Vogt, C.; Eckhof, A.; Witt, I.: Twenty-four-hour pattern of growth hormone secretion in the rhesus monkey: studies including alterations of the sleep/wake and sleep stage cycles. Endocrinology *109:* 513–522 (1981).

2   Quabbe, H.-J.: Search for a primate model of human sleep-related hormone secretion; in Van Cauter, Copinschi, Human pituitary hormones. Circadian and episodic variations, pp. 42–63 (Martinus Nijhoff, The Hague 1981).

3   Jenkins, G. M.; Watts, D. G.: Spectral analysis and its applications (Holden-Day, San Francisco 1968).

4   Quabbe, H.-J.: Chronobiology of growth hormone secretion. Chronobiologia *4:* 217–246 (1977).

5   Quigley, M. E.; Ropert, J. F.; Yen, S. S. C.: Acute prolactin release triggered by feeding. J. clin. Endocr. Metab. *52:* 1043–1045 (1981).

6   Frantz, A. G.: Rhythms in prolactin secretion; in Krieger, Endocrine rhythms, pp. 175–186 (Raven Press, New York 1979).

7   Weeke, J.: Circadian and ultradian variations in serum TSH and thyroid hormones in normal man and in patients with treated and untreated primary hypothyroidism; in Van Cauter, Copinschi, Human pituitary hormones. Circadian and episodic variations, pp. 132–151 (Martinus Nijhoff, The Hague 1981).

H.-J. Quabbe, MD, Section of Endocrinology, Department of Internal Medicine, Klinikum Steglitz, Freie Universität Berlin, Hindenburgdamm 30, D-1000 Berlin 45 (FRG)

Adv. biol. Psychiat., vol. 11, pp. 60–63 (Karger, Basel 1983)

Hormonal Changes after Jet Lag in Normal Man

Daniel Désir[a], *Eve Van Cauter*[a, b], *Samuel Refetoff*[b], *Victor S. Fang*[b], *Jacqueline Golstein*[a], *Michèle Fèvre-Montange*[c], *Marc L'Hermite*[a], *Claude Robyn*[a], *Claude Jadot*[a], *Michèle Szyper*[a], *Jean-Paul Spire*[b], *Pierre Noël*[a], *Georges Copinschi*[a]

[a] Free University of Brussels, Belgium; [b] University of Chicago, Ill., USA; [c] University of Lyons, France

Introduction

Disruption and desynchronization of bodily rhythms have become a common experience for millions of travellers flying each year across time zones. Subjective reports frequently mention symptoms such as tiredness, daytime sleepiness, sleep disturbances and poor physical and mental fitness after abrupt time shifts. As shown in previous studies on the effects on real and simulated flights, rapid transmeridian displacements induce many behavioral and biological changes [1–3]. Since the endocrine system plays a key role in the adaptation to environmental variations, disruptions in the temporal organization of hormone secretion might be involved in the pathogenesis of the jet lag syndrome. The development of sensitive radioassays now allows to measure the concentrations of several plasma hormones on small blood samples withdrawn at frequent intervals throughout the 24-hour span, thus providing detailed data on circadian and episodic profiles of hormone secretion.

In the present study, healthy males were submitted to seven 24-hour investigations over a total period of 10 weeks during a round trip by jet from Brussels to Chicago. Samples of blood were obtained at 15-min intervals during seven 24-hour sessions, and sleep and anxiety and depression scores were recorded. The protocol of the study and a part of hormonal data have already been described in detail elsewhere [4–6].

Subjects and Methods

5 healthy males, aged 21–29 years, were studied. Normality of their physical condition was assessed by an interview, physical and psychiatric examinations and a battery of biological and endocrine tests [4]. Positive factors for selection included emotional stability, adherence to regular social, professional, feeding and sleep schedules and absence of personal or family history of endocrine and psychiatric disease.

The investigation units in Brussels (Belgium) and Chicago (USA) were of similar design. Time zone difference between these locations was 7 h. Except during flights, the subjects adhered constantly to a 16:8 light-dark cycle (lights off from 23.00 to 07.00 h, local time) and received regular meals at 08.00, 12.30 and 19.00 h local time. During travel, they were exposed to the usual conditions of civil air transport and sleep within aircrafts was prevented. Sleep deprivation periods lasted 23 h for the westward flight and 33 h for the eastward flight, owing to the constraints of airline schedules. Study 1 was performed in Brussels after 4 nights of adjustment to the blood sampling and sleep recording procedures. Study 2 began 25 h after arrival in Chicago and studies 3 and 4 were performed 11 and 21 days after arrival. Studies 5, 6 and 7 corresponded to one (33 h), 11 and 21 days after return to Brussels. Sleep was recorded and scored using standard techniques [7]. Details of the blood sampling procedures were given elsewhere [4].

Total plasma proteins were measured in each sample in order to detect a possible plasma dilution resulting from the sampling procedure. 36 out of 3,264 samples were found to be significantly diluted and were discarded [4]. Plasma ACTH, cortisol, melatonin and prolactin were determined on each sample using radioimmunoassays [4, 5].

Psychopathological evaluation of the subjects using Hamilton scales for depression and anxiety [8, 9] were carried out by the same investigator (*C. J.*) throughout the study.

Low frequency (e. g. circadian) components of individual profiles of each blood component were evaluated using a method based on the building of a best-fit pattern [10, 11].

A computer program was also developed to obtain a quantitative evaluation of ultradian (i. e. episodic) oscillations of plasma hormones [10, 11].

Results and Comments

At the present stage of analysis, results of this study can be summarized as follows:

The period of maximal secretion and the quiescent period of the 24-hour pattern of ACTH and cortisol adapted differently to the time shifts, suggesting that the various components of the pituitary-adrenal periodicity may be under different controls. Partial shifts of the acrophase toward the new clock time occurred as early as 1 day after travel in both directions, and the synchronization of the acrophase was completed 10 days after both westward and eastward flights. In contrast, the quiescent period needed at least 3 weeks to adapt to Chicago time (alterations consisted of desynchronisation and fragmentation) but returned to normal on the 11th day after arrival in Brussels.

Jet lag failed to produce quantitative secretory alterations for ACTH, cortisol and prolactin, since no significant changes were observed in the 24-hour mean levels, the amplitude of the circadian rhythms, or the frequency and global magnitude of episodic fluctuations of these hormones. In contrast, decreased 24-hour mean levels of plasma melatonin were observed after the westward shift.

Disruptions in the sleep patterns (with an increase in rapid eye movement sleep) and subjective psychological discomfort (rated by Hamilton's anxiety and depression scales) were highly significant after the eastward flight only. While persistent disruption of the pituitary-adrenal periodicity were observed, sleep and psychological indexes had returned to normal when recorded 11 days after flight, although no consistent correlation was fond between the disturbances of the pituitary-adrenal periodicity and the level of psychological discomfort, subjects with the highest and lowest scores on the Hamilton's scales showing, respectively, the slowest and fastest adaptation of the cortisol acrophase to the new clock time.

Despite an apparent correlation between the melatonin and the cortisol rhythms during the unperturbed state, a lack ot relationship is supported on the basis of discrepancies in adaptation rates of both hormones (abolishment of the 6-hour time difference between melatonin and cortisol rhythms during the period of adaptation after time shifts).

The adaptation of the prolactin (PRL) circadian pattern to jet lag was strikingly similar to that of the pituitary-adrenal periodicity. Both had components adapting in less than 10 days (cortisol major acrophase; PRL 'sleep' acrophase) without westward-eastward difference, and components requiring more than 10 days to adapt to westward shift but less than 10 days to adapt to eastward shift (quiescent period of cortisol secretion; pattern of PRL secretion during wakefulness). An endogenous (non-sleep-dependent) circadian periodicity of plasma PRL was detected in the profiles obtained after the flights, as well as in control studies involving simple sleep deprivation in Brussels, challenging the concept that nighttime PRL rise is purely dependent upon sleep.

The relationship between episodic variations (secretory peaks) of plasma PRL and REM/non-REM cyclicity was shown to be artifactual since episodic PRL fluctuation during sleep occurred at purely random frequency in basal studies as well as in studies performed after transmeridian flights.

Further studies are required to fully delineate the role of alterations in sleep and hormonal secretion in the pathogenesis of the jet lag syndrome and their influence on the associated psychological and behavioral manifestations.

References

1 McFarland, R.A.: Influence of changing time zones on air crews and passengers. Aerospace Med. *45:* 648–658 (1974).
2 Klein, K.E.; Wegmann, H.M.; Hunt, B.I.: Desynchronization of body temperature and performance circadian rhythms as a result of outgoing and home going transmeridian flights. Aerospace Med. *43:* 119–124 (1972).
3 Lafontaine, E.; Lavernhe, J.; Courillon, J.; Medvedeff, M.; Ghata, J.: Influence of air travel east-west and vice-versa on circadian rhythms of urinary elimination of potassium and 17-hydroxy-corticoids. Aerospace Med. *38:* 944–954 (1967).
4 Désir, D.; Van Cauter, E.; Fang, V.S.; Martino, E.; Jadot, C.; Spire, J.P.; Noël, P.; Refetoff, S.; Copinschi, G.; Golstein, J.: Effects of 'jet lag' on hormonal patterns. I. Procedures, variations in total plasma proteins, and disruption of adrenocorticotropin-cortisol periodicity. J. clin. Endocr. Metab. *52:* 628–641 (1981).
5 Fèvre-Montange, M.; Van Cauter, E.; Refetoff, S.; Désir, D.; Tourniaire, J.; Copinschi, G.: Effects of 'jet lag' on hormonal patterns. II. Adaptation of melatonin circadian periodicity. J. clin. Endocr. Metab. *52:* 642–649 (1981).
6 Van Cauter, E.; Refetoff, S.; Désir, D.; Jadot, C.; Fèvre-Montange, M.; Fang, V.S.; Golstein, J.; L'Hermite, M.; Robyn, C.; Noël, P.; Spire, J.P.; Copinschi, G.: Adaptation of 24-hour hormonal patterns and sleep to jet lag; in Van Cauter, Copinschi (eds.), Human pituitary hormones: circadian and episodic variations (Martinus Nijhoff, The Hague 1981).
7 Rechtschaffen, A.; Kales, A.: A manual of standardized terminology, techniques and scoring system for sleep stages in normal subjects (Public Health Service, Government Printing Office, Washington 1968).
8 Hamilton, M.: A rating scale for depression. J. Neurol. Neurosurg. Psychiat. *23:* 56–62 (1960).
9 Hamilton, M.: The assessment of anxiety states by rating. Br. J. med. Psychol. *32:* 50–55 (1959).
10 Van Cauter, E.: Method for characterization of 24-hour temporal variation of blood components. Am. J. Physiol., *E237:* E255–264 (1979).
11 Van Cauter, E.: Quantitative methods for the analysis of circadian and episodic hormone fluctuations; in Van Cauter, Copinschi (eds.), Human pituitary hormones: Circadian and episodic variations (Martinus Nijhoff, The Hague 1981).

Daniel Désir, MD, Free University of Brussels, Hôpital Erasme, Department of Endocrinology, 808 Route de Lennik, B-1070 Brussels (Belgium)

Adv. biol. Psychiat., vol. 11, pp. 64–71 (Karger, Basel 1983)

Professional Activity and Physiological Rhythms[1]

F. Lille, Y. Burnod

Laboratoire de Physiologie du Travail, CNRS, et Laboratoire U3 de l'Inserm, Paris, France

Introduction

In their recent review, *Regal and Connoly* [19] first asserted that there has been remarkably little focus on the interactions between social behavior and biological rhythms, and that human chronobiological studies generally are not concerned with social and temporal conditioning.

Sociological or physiological disturbances occurring during shift work have been known for many years, but it was only in 1978 that *Reinberg* et al. [20], based on a hypothesis by *Aschoff* [1], observed that a small circadian rhythm amplitude for certain variables such as oral temperature, peak expiratory flow and urinary 17-OHCS may be an index of an individual's ability to phase-shift and adjust easily to a new activity/rest schedule. At the same time, the interruption of rhythmic patterns of activity and inactivity has been proposed by *Michon* [15] as a measure of perceptual motor load and by *Chapple* [4] as a measure of severity and length of a stress reaction.

Polyphasic patterns of sleep-wakefulness are characteristic of human infants [10], and *Kleitman* [11] proposed that a basic rest activity cycle (BRAC), expressed at night in REM/non-REM alternation, continues throughout the day. Behavioral ultradian rhythms have been reported during wakefulness, for example in oral activity [5, 6, 18], in motor activity [8], in performance [7, 9, 17], in perceptual illusion [13] or in waking fantasy [12]. In a previous study [3] of university and factory personnel, physiological parameters and behavioral activities measured during 8 regular working

[1] This research has been supported in part by DGRST grant No. 79.7.1434.

hours were found to have synchronized variations at several moments. These variations coincided for all the parameters (EEG, EKG, EOG, EMG) and professional activities, and occurred with an average interval of 93 min (with large inter- and intra-subject differences). They were better individualized in university than in factory personnel. To examine the influence of work stress on these 90 min oscillations the same study was also performed with air traffic controllers during both day and night duty periods. The first results, concerning air traffic controllers' (ATC) heart rate and circadian variations, have been previously published [14].

Material and Methods

Sample Population

Telemetric recordings and behavioral observations were performed on 3 subject groups during their daily occupational activity: 10 factory (F) personnel (9 women and 1 man) with a mean age of 37 ± 4 years; 10 university (U) researchers or teachers (8 women and 2 men) with a mean age of 39 ± 5 years; and 9 air traffic controllers (ATC) with a mean age of 34 ± 8 years.

The F were involved in the production of electronic elements for the aeronautic industry, were all in the same wiring workshop (about 100 people), and had a strict production schedule. Recordings were made continuously from 08.15 to 16.15 even during the 40-min lunch break at 11.40.

The U were also recorded during 8 h but with arrival, departure and lunch hours more variable than those for the F. They freely organized their time to do research in the laboratory, prepare lectures, do administration work and so on.

The ATC volunteered to be recorded at one regional control center, each during a day and a night shift within a 48-hour period. All had been on shift air traffic control from 3 to 30 years. The shift schedule was organized over an 8-day period. All the ATC were recorded continuously during two working periods: the first during shift 3 (from 08.00 until 17.30 with two interruptions for a meal and a coffee break) and the second during shift 4 (6 ATC from 19.00 until 24.00 and 3 from 19.00 until 03.00, without interruption). 50 ATC (two teams of 25) were present concurrently in the control room working at different air sectors.

Techniques

Telemetric recordings were obtained from a 6-channel equipment: one for electrocardiogram (EKG), one for electromyogram from the nape of the neck (EMG), one for electrooculogram (EOG), and three for electroencephalogram (EEG) with electrodes placed on the left frontal, temporal and occipital regions, the reference being on the vertex. Electrodes were attached by flexible wires to a small transmitter worn on the waist thus permitting the subjects under study to move freely and be recorded up to 100 m from the receptor. Two observers continuously noted subject behavior (eating, nibbling, drinking, smoking, speaking, displacements, etc.) and all available information about occupation problems (mainly for ATC: difficulties, number of planes) as well as visits, phone calls, etc.

Analysis of each 20-second period was made: count of heart beats, palpebral blinks, and estimation of EMG on three levels (absent, low amplitude, and high amplitude). To analyze

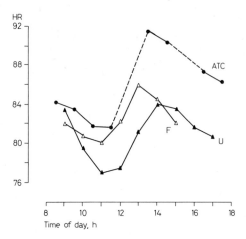

Fig. 1. Mean hourly HR for the 3 different professional groups during the day. ATC = Air traffic controllers; F = factory personnel; U = university personnel.

the EEG recordings three indices from the occipito-vertex derivation were chosen: the alpha-rhythm duration (alpha-index), the theta-rhythm duration (theta-index) and the presence or absence of slow delta-waves.

Data for each 20-second period and each parameter were encoded for statistical analysis on a Modcomp P IV computer. For each subject moments of synchronization were observed taking into account tree or more of six associated variations (decrease of theta-index, increase of alpha-index, increase of number of blinks, drop in muscle tone, heart rate variations, and work activity changes).

Results

Long-Term Variations

Curves of mean hourly heart rate (HR) values were similar for the three professional groups (fig. 1): progressive decrease during the morning with minimal values at about 11.00, increase to the maximal between 13.00 and 14.00, followed by another decrease. Variations were the highest for the ATC especially in the afternoon, and the same HR timing was observed for them during day or night shifts (fig. 2) (correlation coefficient between the two was 0.71).

For the other physiological parameters (EOG, EMG, EEG), such long-term variations were not systematic.

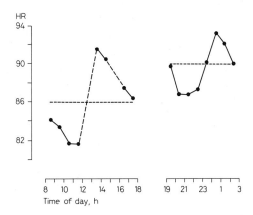

Fig. 2. Mean hourly HR for ATC group during day and night. Dotted lines represent day and night mean values.

Table I. Percentage of occurrence for each parameter variation.

	U	F	ATC	
			day	night
	(n = 49)	(n = 29)	(n = 29)	(n = 30)
EKG	100	86	62	70
EOG	86	83	59	57
EMG	77	96	31	50
?	84	69	72	90
α	43	17	59	30
Activity	80	90	41	63

Short-Term Variations

The number of synchronized moments was greater for U (49) than for F (29) or ATC (29) and varied according to the subject (from 1 to 6). Duration of these moments was similar for the three groups (7–8.5 min). Synchronization of the different parameters was less for ATC than for the two other groups, in particular, simultaneous variations of 5 or 6 criteria were rarely observed for ATC. Table I represents the percentage of occurrence for each parameter variation, and it should be noted that the amplitude variations were smaller for the ATC. Intervals between two consecutive synchronized moments (fig. 3) were 89 ± 43 min for U, 120 ± 77

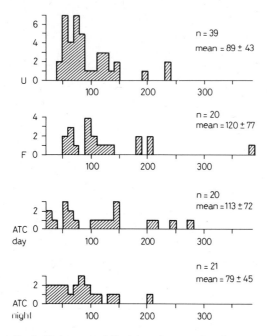

Fig. 3. Histograms of the intervals separating the moments of synchronization.

min for F, 113 ± 72 min during the day and 79 ± 45 during the night for ATC (Student's t test indicated only a significant difference at $p < 0.05$ between U and F). Meal, work or sleep time schedules did not seem to have any influence on the occurrence of the synchronized moments; nonetheless, they were more numerous between 11.00 and 12.00.

Discussion

HR is one of the most intensively measured physiological parameters, and its increase in relation to physical effort is basic in ergonomy. HR circadian changes have been described in many studies [reviewed in ref. 21], but ultradian HR rhythms have been less explored. In this study the same mean hourly HR variation was observed for the three professional groups during the day and for the ATC at night. Same oscillations were observed for each subject. These oscillations, corresponding closely to a work rhythm organized around habitual daily work duration, could be conditioned by one of the most important temporal constraints in the human adult: the professional time schedule. The amplitude of the variation (from 6 to 10 beats/min) during the working period is more important than that described for the circadian oscillation (from 2.5 to 8.5 beats/min). The maximal mean value occurring in the post-prandial period is in part related to the meal but it is also tied to work resumption. In addition, for the ATC 13.00 h corresponds to a period of dense air traffic and therefore stress. But it is interesting to note that for the ATC the maximal measured mean HR value occurred during night work, contrary to shift-work literature.

In contrast to this 8-hour work rhythm, synchronized moments within a shorter time span have important intra- and inter-subject differences. The number of synchronized moments is less important for F and ATC than for U. For the most part, in the ATC group intervals between synchronized moments were extensively variable. So, the question has to be asked whether it represents a rhythm, or, as proposed by *Aschoff* [2] for the alternation between activity and rest, could they be produced on the basis of specific classes of purely stochastic processes. The first descriptions of 90-min cycles were made for isolated subjects and were easier to observe for sleep- or sensory-deprived subjects. In the present study synchronized moments were relatively easier to observe and their occurrence more regular for U working alone in their laboratory than for subjects in a large workshop or a noisy air traffic control room. U can choose freely to interrupt their occupational activities and thus may often be in phase with their endogenous physiological oscillations, thereby reinforcing them. F have a very strict time schedule and have to maintain a steady production level. In contrast, ATC activities are very punctual but transient, and multiple disrupting factors occur; for example, unpredictable changes in plane numbers. If stress can be expressed as being disruptive or interruptive actions or information, air traffic control is dramatically stressful, and the effect of this stress is evident on the HR producing a large increase at randomly distributed epochs. This can be compared to large stress effects which have been described as being able to have a masking effect on the circadian cortisol secretion rhyhtm [16].

In the present study each physiological parameter was found to be influenced differently by environmental events, and any weak physiological coupling not reinforced by the regular periodic work interruptions tended to disappear. Thus, professional activities may within the short-term disrupt weakly coupled 90-min synchronized moments or within the long-term bring about such oscillations as 8-hour HR rhythms.

Summary

Physiological parameters (EEG, EKG, EOG, EMG) and behavioral activities were continuoulsy measured during working hours in university personnel (U), factory workmen (F) and air traffic controllers (ATC). For these 3 occupational groups the same heart rate variations were observed during work periods. Other parameters did not have this rhythm during work, but 'moments' occurred having synchronous variations of three or more physiological indices with mean intervals of about 90 min. Easily observed for U, they were less apparent for F and ATC. The influence of occupational stress is discussed.

References

1   Aschoff, J.: Features of circadian rhythms relevant for the design of shift schedules. Ergonomics *39:* 739–754 (1978).
2   Aschoff, J.: A survey on biological rhythms; in Biological rhythms. Handbook of behavioral neurobiology, vol. 4, pp. 3–10 (Plenum Press, New York 1981).
3   Burnod, Y.; Cheliout, F.; Hazemann, P.; Lille, F.: Synchronisation de différents paramètres physiologiques au cours de la veille chez l'homme. Revue EEG Neurophysiol. *4:* 366–376 (1979).
4   Chapple, E. D.: Experimental production of transients in human interaction. Nature, Lond. *228:* 630–633 (1970).
5   Friedman, S.; Fisher, C.: On the presence of a rhythmic, diurnal, oral instinctual drive cycle in man: a preliminary report. J. Am. psychoanalyt. Ass. *225:* 959–960 (1967).
6   Friedman, S.: On the presence of a variant form of instinctual regression: oral drive cycles in obesity-bulimia. Psychoanalyt. Q. *41:* 364–383 (1972).
7   Globus, G. G.; Drury, E.; Phoebus, E.; Boyd, R.: Ultradian rhythms and performance. Percept. Mot. Skills *33:* 1171–1174 (1971).
8   Globus, G. G.; Phoebus, E.; Humphries, J.; Boyd, R.; Sharp, R.: Ultradian rhythms in human telemetered gross motor activity. Aerospace Med. *44:* 882–887 (1973).
9   Klein, R.; Armitage, R.: Rhythms in human performance: 1½-hour oscillations in cognitive style. Science *204:* 1326–1328 (1979).
10   Kleitman, N.; Engelman, T. G.: Sleep characteristics in infants. J. appl. Physiol. *6:* 269–282 (1953).
11   Kleitman, N.: Sleep and wakefulness, 552 pp. (University of Chicago Press, Chicago 1963).
12   Kripke, D. F.; Sonnenschein, D.: A biologic rhythm in waking fantasy; in The stream of consciousness, pp. 321–332 (Plenum Press, New York 1978).
13   Lavie, P.; Levy, M.; Coolidge, F. L.: Ultradian rhythms in the perception of the spiral after effect. Physiol. Psychol. *3:* 144–146 (1975).
14   Lille, F.; Sens-Salis, D.; Ullsperger, P.; Cheliout, F.; Borodulin, L.; Burnod, Y.: Heart rate variations in air traffic controllers during day and night work; in Night and shift work biological and social aspects. Advances in the biosciences, vol. 30, pp. 391–397 (Pergamon Press, Oxford 1981).
15   Michon, J. A.: Tapping regularity as a measure of perceptual motor load. Ergonomics *9:* 401–412 (1966).

16 Moore-Ede, M.C.; Sulzman, F.M.: Internal temporal order; in Biological rhythms handbook of behavioral neurobiology, vol. 4, pp. 215–241 (Plenum Press, New York 1981).

17 Orr, W.C.; Hoffman, H.J.; Hegge, F.W.: Ultradian rhythms in extended performance. Aerospace Med. *45:* 995–1000 (1974).

18 Oswald, I.; Merrington, J.; Lewis, H.: Cyclical 'on demand' oral intake by adults. Nature, Lond. *225:* 959–960 (1970).

19 Regal, P.J.; Connoly, M.S.: Social influences on biological rhythms. Behaviour *3–4:* 171–199 (1980).

20 Reinberg, A.; Vieux, N.; Ghata, J.; Chaumont, A.J.; Laporte, A.: Is the rhythm amplitude related to the ability to phase-shift circadian rhythms of shift-workers? J. Physiol., Paris *74:* 405–409 (1978).

21 Smolenski, M.H.; Tatar, S.E.; Bergman, S.A.; Losman, J.G.; Barnard, C.N.; Dasco, C.C.; Kraft, I.A.: Circadian rhythmic aspects of human cardiovascular function. A review by chronobiologic statistical methods. Chronobiologia *3:* 337–371 (1976).

F. Lille, MD, Laboratoire de Physiologie du Travail du CNRS, 91, Boulevard de l'Hôpital, F-75013 Paris (France)

Adv. biol. Psychiat., vol. 11, pp. 72–79 (Karger, Basel 1983)

Behavioral Analogs of the REM-nonREM Cycle [1]

D. F. Kripke, P. A. Fleck, D. J. Mullaney, M. L. Levy

Department of Psychiatry, University of California, San Diego, and San Diego Veterans Administration Medical Center, San Diego, Calif., USA

Since *Kleitman* [1] first presented his hypothesis that there is a 'basic rest-activity cycle' (BRAC), several groups have searched for behavioral expressions of this cycle in waking life. Quite a variety of behavioral cycles with periods of about 90 min have been described. For example, *Friedman and Fisher* [2] described a rhythm in oral behaviors. *Globus* [3] and *Globus* et al. [4] reported about-90-min rhythms in the Rorschach responses and in activity. *Lavie* [5] and *Lavie* et al. [6] reported rhythms in the spiral after-effect illusion and in certain performance tasks. *Kripke* [7] found 10 to 20 cycle/day frequencies in EEG measures and in lever presses for water among isolated subjects. *Kripke and Sonnenschein* [8] described such a rhythm in subjective fantasies.

These positive reports must be taken with a grain of salt, because most of these studies (including our own) had rather few subjects, some weaknesses in statistical techniques, and partially equivocal results. In addition, there has been difficulty in replicating some of the results. For example, in further replications in our laboratory, we have not consistently found a 90-min rhythm in fantasies – the spectral peak is closer to one cycle per 180 min when results from about 50 separate subjects are averaged. Some negative findings should also be noted. For example, we found that there is no 90-min rhythm in gross activity itself [9]. Thus, if there are 90-min cycles in some behaviors, gross activity is a poor representative and 'basic rest-activity cycle' is a misnomer. Also, it has been shown that the

[1] Supported in part by ONR N00014-79-C-0317, by the Veterans Administration, and by NIMH RSDA 5 K02 MH00117 (to DFK).

about-90-min cycle in stomach contractions, first reported by *Wada* [10], is not related either to stage REM sleep or to day-time fantasies [11, 12]. Thus, we must consider that there are multiple pacemakers with about the same frequency, and we become obliged to sort out which is which [13].

One of the most intriguing descriptions of 90-min cycles has been the report of *Klein and Armitage* [14], who described a '1½-hour oscillation in cognitive style'. Two simultaneous matching tasks were tested, which were thought to reflect asymmetrical hemispheric specialization. A verbal task required deciding whether pairs consisting of one uppercase and one lowercase letter represented the same letter of the alphabet. A spatial perception task required a decision as to whether pairs of seven-dot random patterns were identical. Responses were recorded with paper and pencil. Each task was performed for 3 min every 15 min for 8 h. 8 young subjects were tested together in a room on a single day and the experimenters were apparently present during the tasks. Spectral peaks were described at frequencies of approximately 1 cycle/96 min in both tasks, however, the 96-min peak was neither the only significant spectral peak nor the most prominent. Performance varied inversely between the tasks. Results were interpreted as suggesting a BRAC-like cycle in hemispheric dominance.

Excited by this report, we decided to repeat the study with certain elaborate precautions including isolation of subjects, computerized testing, and control of motivation.

Methods

11 young volunteers, 3 females and 8 males (aged 18–32) served as subjects. All were students recruited by advertisements. All were right-handed and from right-handed families.

A microcomputer system was employed to present performance tasks, regulate the timing of the performance trials, score performance and reward subjects, and record the results. There were three different tasks and 5 subjective measures during each 10-min interval. First, for 3 min, a letter-matching task with uppercase and lowercase letters was displayed on the computer screen. Subjects worked as rapidly as possible, responding by typing 'S' on the keyboard if the letters were the same and 'D' if they were different. A harsh sound provided negative feedback for errors. Next, for 3 min, pairs of random 7-dot patterns were displayed, some identical and some different, and 'S' and 'D' responses were again required and feedback given. Next, for 3 min a brief automated version of the Wilkinson Auditory Vigilance Task was presented [15]. In the last minute, subjects were asked to give visual-analog self-ratings on sleepiness and attention-fantasy scales and to indicate how much they had had to eat, how much they had had to drink, and whether they had visited the rest room during the prior 10-min interval. Since it was possible to respond to these latter queries within about 15 s, approximately 45 s were provided for rest, snacking, and rest room trips before resumption of the task presentations. Food in snack-sized quantities and non-caffeinated beverages were provided ad libitum, but the task presentation was not halted for eating, drinking, or rest room needs. Drinks were quantified in 30-cm^3 cups and snack foods were assigned arbitrary units.

Subjects were paid $2.00 per hour for participation in the experiment plus up to an additional $2.00 per hour based on the excellence of their performance. After each 3-minute task, and again at the end of each 10 min, the computer informed the subject how much she/he had earned as well as the hourly earning rate achieved. Thus, the computer supplied continuous feedback to maintain the subjects' interest and motivation.

Subjects made an initial visit to the laboratory to learn about the experiment, sign voluntary informed consent, and practice the tasks to familiarize themselves with the experimental setting. A few days later, they returned to the laboratory and worked continuously at the performance tasks for a 10-hour period from approximately 8:00 a.m. to 6:00 p.m. Each subject worked alone in a lighted 3×3.5 m room. Other than brief visits by experimenters to replenish the food and monitor any equipment difficulties, each subject was undisturbed. Subjects were permitted to briefly leave the laboratory to visit the rest room.

Six scores for each performance were obtained each hour, or 60 over the course of each 10-hour experiment. To examine for rhythmic processes, the means from each time series were removed and the autocorrelation functions and hanned spectral transforms computed with a spectral resolution of 0, 4.6, 9.2, 14.4, 18.0 ... 64.4 cycles/day [16]. A spectral peak at one cycle/100 min or 14.4 cycles/day was prospectively predicted. For the group of subjects, the mean and confidence limits of the individual spectra were computed for each variable. Product-moment correlations among variables were also computed.

Results

Most subjects performed steadily and relatively consistently throughout the study. It was necessary to excuse 1 male subject when it was discovered that he was taking frequent breaks from the tasks and not complying with the protocol. Thus data for 10 subjects were analyzed. Subjects performed the Wilkinson Auditory Vigilance Task without error in the majority of 3-min test intervals, so these data could not be analyzed for changes over time.

The letter-matching and dot-matching tasks were substantially correlated. Taking the z-transform of r (the product-moment correlation coefficient) to obtain the mean for the group, an average positive correlation of $r = 0.59$ was found ($t = 5.90$, $p < 0.002$ for the mean correlation). Neither the sleepiness nor fantasy ratings were significantly correlated with either dot-matching or letter-matching. Rest room trips had a small negative correlation with letter-matching, only ($r = -0.25$, $t = 2.24$, $p < 0.05$), but obviously could not account for much covariance. Eating and drinking were not significantly correlated with either task performance.

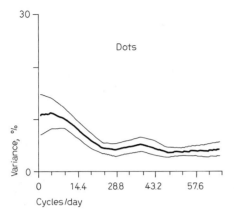

Fig. 1. Mean of 10 spectra for 10 subjects, surrounded by its 95 % confidence limit, is shown for the number of dot pairs matched correctly. The ordinate is the percent of the total variance in each frequency band.

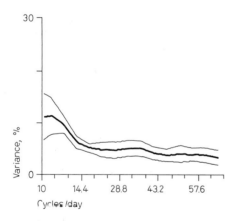

Fig. 2. The mean spectrum for letter pairs matched correctly.

    Plots of the performance and subjective responses of each subject showed no impressive cyclicity in the range of 80–120 min in any measure. The spectra for letter-matching and dot-matching peaked in the 4.8 cycles/ day band (1 cycle/300 min) and dropped off rapidly at higher frequencies (fig. 1, 2). The spectrum for the ratio of letter-matching to dot-matching performance, representing the relative performance in the two tasks, also peaked at 4.8 cycles/day, but the spectral variance was as great in the

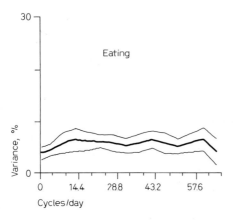

Fig. 3. The mean spectrum for the quantity of eating.

slowest frequency band (0–2.9 cycles/day). The spectra for sleepiness and the attention-fantasy scale also peaked in the 0–2.9 cycles/day band. For both eating and rest room trips, the spectra were rather flat, and there was no frequency significantly exceeding the expectation for random variance, however, the greatest spectral amplitudes were in the 14.4 cycles/day frequency band (1 cycle/84–124 min). The spectrum for eating is shown in figure 3. A substantial peak in drinking behaviors was noted in the 9.6 cycles/day band, significantly exceeding random variance but not significantly exceeding the variance in the adjacent 14.4 cycles/day band.

Discussion

These results fail to confirm the results of *Klein and Armitage* [14]. They lend no support whatsoever to the hypothesis that there is an about-90-min cycle in performances modulated by alternating hemispheric dominance.

Quite a few possibilities might have caused the inconsistency between our results and those of *Klein and Armitage* [14]. Our computer presentation of the tasks must have somewhat altered the speed of responding to the letter- and dot-matching tasks. Our demand characteristics were quite different, since we supplied immediate feedback and monetary rewards. Our model placed much more pressure on the subjects, allowing almost no rest, and each subject was socially isolated. Also, our spectral method was quite conservative. In contrast, since all of *Klein and Armitage's* [14] subjects worked in the same room, it is conceivable that group interactions (e. g., at lunch) or interactions with the experimenters might have biased the results and degraded the independence of subjects. Since these authors found that 3 of 15 tested spectral frequencies were significant, the 96-min frequency was not the most prominent, and the other frequencies found were not predicted a priori, there is some doubt whether their statistical approach yields a conservative estimate of rhythm detection. A most striking disparity was in the relative performance on the dot-matching and letter-matching tasks, where *Klein and Armitage* [14] found inversely varying performances and we found positively correlated performances. It would thus appear that these measures are quite situationally sensitive, which raises doubt as to their generalizability as measures of hemispheric dominance.

It is interesting that we found some weak evidence for cycles at frequencies of 9.6–14.4 cycles/day in eating and drinking behaviors. Cycles in eating and drinking have been reported in several human isolation experiments [2, 7, 17], and rather similar cycles have been described in primates both in isolation and in social-living models [18–21]. Perhaps the similarity of frequency of the primate cycles is surprising, since the REM-non-REM-cycle frequencies of monkeys are about twice those of human adults. Enteric contraction cycles are more similar in frequency among species than are their REM-non-REM cycles [22], which provides another indication that enteric contraction cycles and REM cycles originate from different pacemakers. Since feeding cycles, like enteric contraction cycles, seem rather stable in frequency across species, feeding cycles are more likely to be related to enteric contraction cycles than to REM-non-REM cycles.

The possible rhythm noted in rest room trips was not convincing, both because the spectral peak was insignificant and because this measure was highly discontinuous. Nevertheless, it is interesting to note that urinary excretion volumes have been reported to show similar cycles [23]. Urinary excretion cycles are also not strictly associated with the REM-non-REM cycle [24].

In summary, this experiment was rather negative as regards the hypothesized waking rhythm in hemispheric dominance. Only very weak support was found for previously described rhythms in eating and drinking. Over the years, impressive difficulties have arisen in finding replicable behavioral expressions of the hypothesized BRAC. There seems to be sufficient evidence that some sorts of cyclicity are found in waking humans, on the other hand, these cycles are neither so regular nor so replicable as the BRAC theory might suggest. The cyclic behaviors which have been described seem quite sensitive to situational factors and small variations in experimental designs. At the present time, extreme caution is needed in generalizing about 90 to 100-min cycles in human behavior.

Summary

About-90-min cycles in various waking behaviors have been described, including a 90-min alternation in hemispheric dominance. To confirm this finding, 11 healthy young subjects were isolated for 10 h. Letter-matching and spatial dot-matching tasks were administered every 10 min, while sleepiness, fantasy, eating, and drinking were also monitored. No about-90-min cycle in letter-matching, dot-matching, or their ratio was found, but weak evidence appeared for cycles in eating, drinking, and rest room trips.

References

1   Kleitman, N.: Sleep and wakefulness; 2nd ed. (University of Chicago Press, Chicago 1963).

2   Friedman, S.; Fisher, C.: On the presence of a rhythmic, diurnal, oral instinctual drive cycle in man: a preliminary report. J. Am. psychoanal. Ass. *15:* 317–343 (1967).

3   Globus, G. G.: Observations on sub-circadian rhythms. Psychophysiology *4:* 366 (1968).

4   Globus, G. G.; Phoebus, E. C.; Humphries, J.; Boyd, R.; Sharp, R.: Ultradian rhythms in human telemetered gross motor activity. Aerospace Med. *44:* 882–887 (1973).

5   Lavie, P.: Ultradian rhythms in the perception of two apparent motions. Chronobiology *3:* 214–218 (1976).

6   Lavie, P.; Gopher, D.; Zohar, D.; Gonen, A.: Ultradian rhythms in prolonged human performance. Final technical report for grant No. DA-ERO-77-G-057 (Technion-Israel Institute of Technology, Technion City, Haifa 1978).

7   Kripke, D. F.: An ultradian biological rhythm associated with perceptual deprivation and REM sleep. Psychosom. Med. *34:* 221–234 (1972).

8   Kripke, D.; Sonnenschein, D.: A biologic rhythm in waking fantasy; in Pope, Singer, The stream of consciousness, pp. 321–332 (Plenum, New York 1978).

9   Kripke, D. F.; Mullaney, D. J.; Wyborney, V. G.; Messin, S.: There's no basic rest-activity cycle; in Stott, Raftery, Sleight, Goulding, ISAM 1977. Proc. 2nd Int. Symp. on Ambulatory Monitoring (Academic Press, London 1978).

10 Wada, T.: An experimental study of hunger and its relation to activity. Archs Psychol. Monogr. *8:* 1 (1922).

11 Lavie, P.; Kripke, D. F.; Hiatt, J. F.; Harrison, J.: Gastric rhythms during sleep. Behav. Biol. *23:* 526–530 (1978).

12   Hiatt, J. F.; Kripke, D. F.; Lavie, P.: Relationships among psychophysiologic ultradian rhythms. Chronobiology, suppl. 1, pp. 30 (1975).
13   Kripke, D. F.: Ultradian rhythms in behavior and physiology; in Brown, Graeber, Rhythmic aspects of behavior, pp. 313–343 (Erlbaum, Hillsdale 1982).
14   Klein, R.; Armitage, R.: Rhythms in human performance: 1½-hour oscillations in cognitive style. Science 204: 1326–1328 (1979).
15   Wilkinson, R. T.: Sleep deprivation: performance tests for partial and selective sleep deprivation. Prog. clin. Psychol. 8: 28–43 (1969).
16   Jenkins, G. B.; Watts, D. G.: Spectral analysis and its applications (Holden-Day, New York 1968).
17   Oswald, I. L.; Merrington, J.; Lewis, H.: Cyclical 'on demand' oral intake by adults. Nature, Lond. 225: 959–960 (1970).
18   Bowden, D. M.; Kripke, D. F.; Wyborney, V. G.: Ultradian rhythms in waking behavior of rhesus monkeys. Physiol. Behav. 21: 929–933 (1978).
19   Delgado-Garcia, J. M.; Grau, C.; DeFeudis, P.; Del Pozo, F.; Jimenez, J. M.; Delgado, J. M. R.: Ultradian rhythms in the mobility and behavior of rhesus monkeys. Expl Brain Res. 25: 79–91 (1976).
20   Delgado, J. M. R.; Del Pozo, F.; Montero, P.; Monteagudo, J. L.; O'Keeffe, T.; Kline, N. S.: Behavioral rhythms of gibbons on Hall's Island. J. interdisc. Cycle Res. 9: 147–168 (1978).
21   Maxim, P. E.; Bowden, D. M.; Sackett, G. P.: Ultradian rhythms of solitary and social behavior in rhesus monkeys. Physiol Behav. 17: 337–344 (1976).
22   Ruckebush, Y.; Bueno, L.: Electrical spiking activity of the small intestine as an ultradian rhythm. Proc. Int. Congr. Physiol., vol. 12, p. 789 (1977).
23   Lavie, P.; Kripke, D. F.: Ultradian rhythms in urine flow in waking humans. Nature, Lond. 269: 142–143 (1977).
24   Luboshitzky, R.; Lavie, P.; Soik, Y.; Glick, S. M.; Leroith, D.; Shen-Orr, Z.; Barzilai, D.: Antidiuretic hormone secretion and urine flow in aged catheterized patients. Technion Inst. Technol. J. Life Scis 8: 99–103 (1978).

D. F. Kripke, MD, Department of Psychiatry (116), V. A. Medical Center,
3350 La Jolla Village Drive, San Diego, CA 92161 (USA)

Adv. biol. Psychiat., vol. 11, pp. 80–94 (Karger, Basel 1983)

Neurobehavioural Organization at Early Age and Risk for Psychopathology

Alex F. Kalverboer[1]

Laboratory for Experimental Clinical Psychology, Groningen, The Netherlands

Introduction

It is not surprising that in humans the importance of behavioural periodicity for adaptation to the external environment was firstly taken into account with respect to the earliest phases of extrauterine life. At this age, the alternation of sleep-wake states strongly dominates, whereas periodicity characterizes biologically essential behaviours, such as sucking and crying. Such behavioural patterns play an important role in early interactions with the social environment. There is strong evidence that the infant's social partners adapt their behaviour to these periodic aspects of the young infant's behavioural repertoire [*Papoušek and Papoušek,* 1983]. Consequently, a lack of consistency in early behavioural organization may play a role in the development of problems in social interaction and contribute to the risk for psychopathology. This is the main thesis of this paper.

Early Risk for Psychopathology

Controversy and confusion characterize literature on 'early risk for psychopathology'. In *retrospective* studies, as reviewed by *Bellak* [1978], almost unanimously more pre- and perinatal complications, such as anoxia, hypoxia, dysmaturity and prematurity at birth, and more early neurological

---

[1] I am grateful to Mrs. G. van Fucht for her help in the preparation of the manuscript and to L. Leartouwer, who drew the figures.

dysfunctions are reported in later psychiatric conditions, such as in schizophrenics, than in controls. On the other hand, in *prospective* studies, no substantial relationships have been found between so-called early risk factors and psychopathology at later age [*Sameroff and Chandler,* 1975]. As far as well-controlled follow-up studies are available, they indicate that associations between signs of early non-optimality and neurobehavioural outcome at a later age are weak to negligible [*Kalverboer,* 1975, 1979]; if reported, they are difficult to cross-validate.

Evidently, in humans the prognostic value of isolated risk factors for neurobehavioural functioning of individuals at a later age is very low. Such factors may be considered as 'surface phenomena', the significance of which depends on their relationship to the child's neurobehavioural organization and its interaction with the environment. This is suggested by a variety of studies which show that the effects of early obstetrical and neurological risk factors for later development strongly depend on the socio-economic conditions in which the individual grows up [*Werner* et al., 1971; *De Ferreira,* in press]. Early non-optimal signs, which have a negligible effect on children's cognitive and social development in higher socio-economic classes, have a significant effect on mental development in children who live in less favourable economic conditions. However, insight in the mechanisms that may determine these differences is completely lacking. Many authors postulate a 'biological vulnerability' factor which, in interaction with environmental factors, should explain differences in outcome [*Tinbergen and Tinbergen,* 1972; *Hamilton,* 1976]. Some recent studies on so-called risk groups can help to specify this rather vague conception.

One is reported by *Marcus* [1981] on the development of infants born to schizophrenics. 13 of 19 infants born to schizophrenics showed poor motor and sensorimotor performance in the first days of extrauterine life and throughout the first year. 7 of these infants also had low-normal birthweights. Further, they were more vulnerable to external insults. The author concluded that these children may have suffered from 'genetically determined' neuro-integrative deficits which may make them more prone to a pathological development. Similarly sized subgroups with identical neuro-integrative impairments have been identified in the offspring of schizophrenics in different populations. Such analyses of individual differences seem to lend support to the idea of a (genetically determined) vulnerability as an important determinant of later outcome. However, independent evidence of any specific neurogenetic deficit is usually lacking.

Moreover, there is great variability in outcome, which may, at least partly, be determined by differences in the quality of the caretaker environment.

One might speculate, as *Marcus* [1981] does, that infants with so-called neuro-integrative deficits were born to those schizophrenic parents who had a neurological impairment themselves. However, one can imagine that such a 'neuro-integrative deficit' will only be a risk factor for the development of clinical schizophrenia in interaction with other, as yet undefined, environmental variables.

A tentative model for such a development has been presented by *Hamilton* [1976]. He suggests that the central mechanism in the pathogenesis of schizophrenia is an interaction between a physiologically based lack of integrative capacities of the organism and informational overload in the (social) environment. Such a model may have a certain heuristic value. However, up till now, direct evidence for such mechanisms in the genesis of psychopathology, i. e. schizophrenia, is lacking. Evidently, simple linear models are insufficient for the explanation of differences in later behavioural outcome. Only precise prospective and retrospective studies can throw some more light on these complex relationships.

Some Sequelae of Early Neurological Complications

This is also indicated in follow-up studies, executed in the Department of Developmental Neurology in Groningen [*Kalverboer,* 1975, 1979], on implications of pre- and perinatal complications for children's neuro-behavioural status at later age. In one project, focus was on the relationships between early obstetrical and neurological 'risk' factors on the one hand and, on the other, neurology and behaviour at preschool and school age. The study concerned a so-called 'low risk sample'; primary criteria for the selection of subjects were 38–42 weeks of gestation, birthweight over 2,500 g and no severe neurological disorder diagnosed during the first months of extrauterine life. Apart from an obstetrical risk score and a neonatal neurological optimality score [*Prechtl,* 1968], scores on two neonatal neurological syndromes, namely hyperexcitability and apathy, were obtained from each of 150 children, 75 boys and 75 girls (table I). Detailed scores on 'free-field' behaviour were obtained at preschool age, whereas teacher's reports (standard questionnaires) provided information on children's school performance and task orientation at the age of 8 [for details see *Kalverboer,* 1975, 1979].

Table I. Classification of neonatal syndromes

---

1. Hyperexcitability syndrome
   a) Moro: low threshold
   b) Tremor: high amplitude, low frequency
   c) Biceps reflex: very exaggerated contraction going on to clonus or
      Knee-jerk reflex: exaggerated response with at least a few beats of clonus
2. Apathy syndrome
   The following responses are absent or of low intensity: recoil of the arms; rooting; sucking; palmar grasp reflex; plantar grasp reflex; labyrinthine reflexes; head lift in prone

---

Definitions and coding according to *Prechtl and Beintema* [1964].

In general, relationships between obstetrical risk and neonatal neurological non-optimality, on the one hand, and neurological and behavioural scores at preschool and school age, on the other, were negligible. Only in a subgroup of 57 boys, without interval complications between birth and preschool age, a significant correlation of 0.28 (p < 0.03) was found between neonatal neurology and neurology at preschool age. Such a low correlation does not allow for any prediction on individual children.

Some intriguing relationships were found between scores in the two neonatal syndromes, apathy and hyperexcitability, on the one hand, and directly observed free-field behaviour at preschool age and teacher's reports at the age of 8, on the other.

Boys who were hyperexcitable in the neonatal neurological examination (n = 9) played longer and at a higher level (p < 0.05) at preschool age than optimal controls. Teachers reported a *better* task orientation in hyperexcitable boys than in optimal controls (p < 0.05). Such differences were not found in girls, These favourable behavioural findings in the hyperexcitable boys are particularly intriguing because this group is generally considered to be at risk for problem behaviour. Detailed inspection of the data strongly suggested that quite a few of the so-called hyperexcitables were in fact healthy newborns, characterized by vigorous lifely motor reactions to weak stimuli. Evidently, the specific hyperexcitability criteria (low threshold Moro, high amplitude tremor, etc.) were not sufficient for unequivocal discrimination between healthy children and children 'at risk' for later problems. The finding suggests that specific neurological signs can only be interpreted if the child's neurobehavioural organization as a whole is taken into account.

Apathetics (n = 22) showed less exploratory activity (p < 0.05) and more contact behaviour (p < 0.02) in a novel room together with the mother than optimal controls, less constructive play (p < 0.03) and longer periods of inactivity (p < 0.05). At 8 years of age apathetic boys had slightly lower task orientation scores than optimal controls (p < 0.10). These follow-up findings in the apathetics at preschool age are rather similar to those commonly reported as signs of the childhood depression syndrome [*Watson*, 1977]. The findings suggest a 'lack of initiative' in apathetics which may in essence be a motivational problem. This is a core phenomenon in *Seligman's* [1975] conception of 'learned helplessness', in which 'reactive depression' is related to an impairment of the development of 'perception of control'. We shall return to this model.

Periodicity and Early Interaction: Models and Preliminary Observations

Linear models, which fail to take social environmental variables into account, are too simple for the explanation of consequences of early somatic risk factors. Transactional models are required which take into account the complex relationship between the infant's behavioural pattern on the one hand and environmental stimulation on the other. Further insight into the mechanisms of deviant development can only be obtained in close follow-up studies, in which the development of interactions and relationships are thoroughly analyzed. Such an attempt has been made in a series of observational studies at the Laboratory for Experimental Clinical Psychology on implications of neonatal neurological disorders for early social interaction. In the following section, I will briefly report on a pilot study of 7 mother-infant pairs during successive breast feedings in the first week after birth. In this pilot study only infants with an optimal neurological condition were included [*Alberts, Kalverboer and Hopkins*, 1983].

In these studies, focus is on the significance of periodicity in the infant's behavioural organization for the interaction with the caretaker. More specifically the question is: is there any relationship between the temporal organization of the baby's sucking behaviour and the temporal organization of tactile stimulation by the mother. The basic idea is that interactions between the organism and the social environment cannot be unterstood in terms of a simple S-R model; the structure of the environment as well as the organization of the behaviour have to be taken into consideration. A short discussion of a learning model and a biopsychological model for the development of psychopathology will lead us to the rationale of the present study.

Seligman's 'Learned Helplessness' Model

The basic idea in *Seligman's* [1975] model is that exposure to uncontrollable, biologically significant events in early phases of life may lead to a condition of 'chronic lack of initiative' at a later age. In pathological form this is one of the cue phenomena in 'reactive depression'. The theoretical concept of 'learned helplessness' has been proposed to account for this effect. The intermediate mechanism is a lack of perceived contingency between the individual's behaviours and their consequents. Experiments in rats and dogs, in which problem-solving behaviour of subjects was observed after exposure to uncontrollable events (generally unavoidable shocks), give some support to the model.

Some effects of non-contingent stimulation on instrumental activity ('head turning at a mobile that turned periodically in a manner unrelated to the infant's behaviour') could be shown in young human infants. However, very little has been understood until now of mechanisms and limitations. Still there are no clear indications that, in humans, the experience of non-contingent stimulation is an important factor in the etiology of reactive depressions.

Experiments in the social learning tradition have exclusively focussed on the manipulation of *environmental factors* which might affect the perception of control: they are generally concerned with the time interval between behaviours of individuals and their consequents, in particular the consistency of the temporal relationship between actions and effects. Characteristics of the organism, which could have an effect on its capacity to perceive contingencies, have not been taken into consideration. However, organisms largely differ with respect to their ability to *perceive* contingencies between their own behaviour and environmental events. The crucial process is 'operant learning', which must be considered to depend on an interaction between the subject's own activity and the patterning of reinforcement from the environment.

Watson's 'Biopsychological' Model

Watson [1977] made an important contribution to this discussion, by paying attention to which *organismic* variables may contribute to the development of 'perception of control'. He argued that 'the most basic adaptive capacity of animate life is the ability to alter behaviour in the service of either increasing or decreasing one's probable contact with biologically significant events. It would seem that when this capacity is thwarted most animals and humans enter a pathological state of diminished behavioural initiative and emotional disturbance.' In *Watson's* [1977] opinion full understanding of possible determinants of depression will require taking account of all the variables that contribute to the perception of control in childhood. Some of the organismic risk factors he mentions are: lower memory capacities to span delays (short term) and for recognizing recurrences (long term), limited or inappropriate attentional functions and poor response rate (producing dysfunctional distribution of practice). All these factors may adversely affect the likelihood that an existing contingency would be accurately perceived. *Watson* [1977] continues: 'nevertheless, virtually no information is available on how these masking factors work individually or interactively to produce interference effects in either the laboratory or the outer world'. Rightly enough, he argues that 'much further research of both the experimental and observational varieties will be needed'. He continues 'particularly useful would be (observational) studies that can inform us of the timing characteristics of contingent and non-contingent stimulation during childhood. Direct observations of human newborns in real life interactions will be required.'

An important 'organismic' factor, not explicitly mentioned by *Watson* [1977], seems to be the organization of the young infant's behaviour, as manifested in sleep-wake cycles and in the periodicity of biologically significant behaviours such as sucking and crying. *Prechtl* [1974] considered the regulation of the behavioural states as a fundamental function of the central nervous system. There is strong evidence from studies in developmental neurology that the reactions of young infants to environmental stimuli are state-related [*Prechtl*, 1974]. Consequently, instability in the temporal organization of behavioural states does affect the consistency of the organism's reactions and, therefore, interferes with a smooth adaptation to the external environment. Such an instability is typically found in children with minor cerebral dysfunctions in the first 2 years of life [*Touwen*, 1976] and at preschool and school age [*Kalverboer*, 1975], and has been reported in newborns [*Prechtl and Beintema*, 1964]. Inconsistency in behavioural organization is the most common finding in children with minor neurological handicaps. It concerns body processes, behavioural states, specific orienting reactions, the organization of movements and body postures, as well as the patterning of complex behaviours during play and social interactions. It can be postulated that selection and processing of information will be less stable and effective in such children than in children with a stable behavioural organization; they will have more problems with the perception of consistent relationships between their own behaviour and its consequences, such that processes of operant learning, for which a stable behavioural organization is required, will be less efficient than in children with an optimal neurological status.

It will be more difficult for the social partner (e.g. the caretaker) to contingently adapt his behaviour to the behaviour of the infant. This is confirmed in clinical reports by mothers of newborns with minor cerebral dysfunctions. Such children reacted unpredictably during interactional activities such as feeding and dressing and many mothers reported that they felt irritated during such interactions [*Prechtl,* 1963]. Furthermore, such children could not easily adapt their behaviour to sleeping and feeding schedules. It is not unlikely that such children run a relatively high risk for the development of emotional problems, such as described by *Watson* [1977] and *Seligman* [1975]. The present studies on mother-infant interaction are based on these considerations. In this pilot study we are particularly interested in 'the variety of the normal'; therefore, only children with an optimal neurological status are included. Focus is on the question: How does the temporal patterning of mother's tactile stimulation of the infant during feeding relate to the temporal organization of the infant's sucking behaviour? Our further observational studies will focus on the effects of neurological syndromes, such as apathy and hyperexcitability on early social interaction and their implications for emotional and social development.

Procedure

Video-recordings were made of 7 mother-infant pairs during breast-feeding. During registrations mother and baby were lying on a bed in a separate room in the obstetric clinic; every attempt was made to minimally interfere with the usual feeding procedure. Two cameras were used; one camera gave an overview of mother and baby, the other a close-up of the section of the image, in which the face of the baby and the breast of the mother were visible. First registrations were made during the second feeding after birth (in this text called 'the early feeding'); they were continued until the sixth to the ninth feeding (in this text called 'the later feeding'). The following behaviours were scored from video-recordings: *in the baby,* sucking bouts and pauses, general body movements, changes in

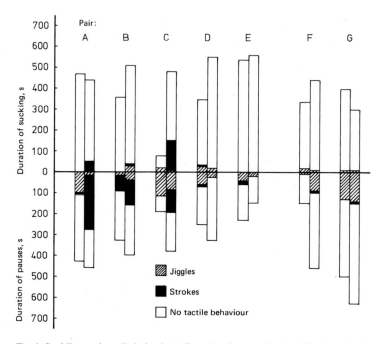

Fig. 1. Suckling and tactile behaviour. Duration in seconds of sucking bouts and sucking pauses of the baby and tactile behaviour (jiggles and strokes) of the mother. For each mother-infant pair the earliest and the latest feedings are represented.

behavioural state, and *in the mother,* frequency and timing of tactile stimulation of the baby. In the mother a distinction was made between two types of tactile stimulation: 'jiggling' and 'stroking' (another category, 'touching', occurred very rarely and was combined with the category 'stroking'). Details of scoring are given in *Alberts, Kalverboer and Hopkins* [1983].

Results

In each baby's sucking behaviour a distinct bout-pause pattern can be observed from the earliest feeding onward. However, there are great interindividual differences in lengths and variability of bouts and pauses (fig. 1–3).

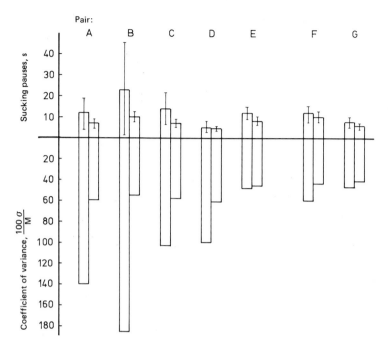

Fig. 2. Pauses in sucking. At the top: duration of sucking pauses (mean ± SD). For each mother-infant pair the earliest and the latest feedings are represented. At the bottom: corrected variances.

In all babies there is a change from early to later feedings, in that sucking *pauses* become shorter and of a more constant length (fig. 2). This is not true for sucking *bouts* which generally remain of similar length over successive feedings (fig. 3). Evidently, behaviour becomes more stable in the course of the first week; this is also suggested by a correlation between bout and pause lengths found in the later and not in the earlier feedings.

Also in the mother's tactile stimulation pattern a distinct bout-pause pattern can be observed. Such a pattern is already visible in the mother's behaviour before the infants starts sucking. Each of the mothers displays an 'individually characteristic' jiggling pattern in the period before the infant starts drinking. However, as soon as sucking starts, the jiggling pattern of the mother adapts to the bout-pause pattern of the baby: in each mother-infant pair and in almost all feedings (13 of 14) the relative amount of tactile behaviour of the mother is much higher during sucking pauses than during

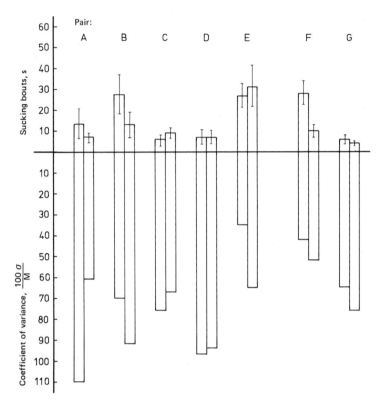

Fig. 3. Sucking bouts. At the top: duration of sucking bouts (mean ± SD). For each pair the earliest and the latest feedings are represented. At the bottom: corrected variances.

sucking bouts (table II). This is found in early as well as in later feedings for both categories of tactile stimulation. After breastfeeding, the pattern of tactile stimulation usually shifts back in the direction of the temporal pattern before drinking started [*Vlaar and Alberts,* 1980]. These observations give support to the idea that pauses in sucking behaviour have a specific significance for the temporal organization of the mother's behaviour during breastfeeding. However, tactile stimulation also occurs during sucking bouts. This is observed slightly more during later than during earlier feedings. Patterns of 'alternation' between babies and mothers as well as patterns of 'simultaneous action' are observed in the mother-infant dialogue.

Table II. Percentage tactile behaviour during sucking pauses

	Pair and feeding													
	A		B		C		D		E		F		G	
	early	late	early	late	early	late	early	late	early	late	early	late	early	late
Pause duration, % of total feeding time	47	51	48	44	71	44	42	37	30	17	31	51	56	68
Duration of jiggles during pauses, % of total jiggle time	97	74	96	60	84	92	68	57	92	79	22	91	92	95

Tactile stimulation by the mother (jiggling) during sucking pauses, relative to the total duration of such pauses (percentages of total feeding time).

Discussion

Discrepancies between results of retrospective studies in adults with manifest psychopathology, and prospective studies on specific risk factors suggest that 'risk for psychopathology' is a most complex concept. Main effect models and simple interaction models are unsuited for the understanding of the contribution of early characteristics of organism and environment to the outcome at later age. One can agree with *Dunn's* [1976] statement: 'The developmental outcome for any particular child is part of a giant equation, with social conditions, the child's temperament, health, mother's sensitivity and style of caretaking, the child's social experiences with others all of potential importance. The internal relationships between these variables are very complicated, and we are just beginning to tease apart the inter-relations between some of these factors, given that others are constant.'

Situations have to be defined in terms of 'psychologically relevant' dimensions, whereas global concepts, such as 'neuro-integrative deficit' and 'caretaking environment' have to be operationalized in terms of characteristics of the infant's and caretaker's behavioural repertoire.

Close follow-up studies in precisely defined samples of children and mothers are required to gain more insight in the mechanisms at work in early neurobehavioural and social development. First results of an observational study of this kind were presented. In the healthy children included in this study, behavioural periodicity of the newborn had a clearcut structuring effect on the behaviour of the mother. Evidently, in the interaction with the healthy infant, the mother needs very little experience to adapt her reactions to the newborn's behaviour. Furthermore, the temporal organization of sucking behaviour stabilized in the course of successive feedings, as was indicated by a more constant length of sucking pauses and the correlation between the lengths of sucking bouts and pauses in later feedings, which was lacking in the early feedings. Such a stabilization makes it more easy for the mother to contingently adapt her own behaviour to temporal aspects of the behaviour of the newborn. However, although there is a growing amount of literature in which the importance of disorders in early behavioural organization for cognitive and social development is stressed [*Trevarthen,* 1974; *Bower,* 1974; *Papoušek and Papoušek,* 1983], nothing is yet known about the impact of a lack of stability/consistency in the baby's behavioural output for cognitive and social development.

Carefully designed follow-up studies are required on precisely defined 'risk samples'. Such studies are in progress in the Laboratory for Experimental Clinical Psychology in Groningen on the implications of neonatal 'hyperexcitability' and 'apathy' syndromes for early social interaction. The rationale of these studies is that a lack of stability of the young infant's behavioural organization may affect information processing and the quality of social interaction with the caretaker. They can help in understanding reciprocal relationships between the developing organism and the caretaker.

'However, the idea that there are two sets of variables, child's characteristics and parent's caretaking style, to be identified early on and from which outcome might be predicted, is far too simple and misleading' [*Dunn*, 1976]. This is certainly true. However, experimental reduction is necessary to gain some insight into the impact of early organismic and environmental factors for later outcome. In particular rhythmical aspects of behaviour may affect the adaptation to social and non-social tasks. In very young, and even more in older children, the role of behavioural periodicity for cognitive and social functioning has been neglected. This is partly due to the dominating position of classical learning theory for the explanation of disorders. One-sided learning models should be replaced by biopsychological models, which account for the importance of periodic aspects of behaviour for coping with environmental demands. Studies, based on such models, may help in clarifying some of the present mysteries with respect to the concept of 'early risk for psychopathology'.

References

Alberts, F.; Kalverboer, A. F., Hopkins, B.: Mother-infant dialogue in the first days of life: an observational study during breast feeding. J. Child Psychol. Psychiat. *24:* 145–161 (1983).

Bellak, L.: Psychiatric aspects of minimal brain dysfunction in adults (Grune & Stratton, New York 1978).

Bower, T. G. R.: Development of infant behavior. Br. med. Bull. *30:* 175–178 (1974).

De Ferreira, M. C. R.: Interactions of nutrition and socio-cultural conditions and their effect on mental development (in press).

Dunn, J.: How far do early differences in mother-child relations affect later development?; in Bateson, Hinde, Growing points in ethology (Cambridge University Press, Cambridge 1976).

Hamilton, V.: Cognitive development in the neuroses and schizophrenias; in Hamilton, Vernon, The development of cognitive processes, pp. 681–731 (Academic Press, London 1976).

Kalverboer, A. F.: A neurobehavioural study in pre-school children. Clinics in developmental medicine, No. 54 (Spastics International Medical Publications / Heinemann Medical Books, London 1975).

Kalverboer, A. F.: Neurobehavioural findings in preschool and school-aged children in relation to pre- and perinatal complications; in Shaffer, Dunn, The first year of life, pp. 55–67 (Wiley, New York 1979).

Marcus, J.: Infants at risk for schizophrenia. The Jerusalem infant development study. Archs gen. Psychiat. *38:* 703–713 (1981).

Papoušek, H.; Papoušek, M.: Biological basis of social interactions: implications of research for the insight in behavioural deviance. J. Child Psychol. Psychiat. *24:* 117–129 (1983).

Prechtl, H. F. R.: The mother-child interaction in babies with minimal brain damage (a follow-up study); in Foss, Determinants of infant behaviour, vol. II (Methuen, London 1963).

Prechtl, H. F. R.: Neurological findings in newborn infants after pre- and perinatal complications; in Jonxis, Visser, Troelstra, Aspects of prematurity and dysmaturity (Kroese, Leiden 1968).

Prechtl, H. F. R.: The behavioural states of the newborn infant (a review). Brain Res. *76:* 185–212 (1974).

Prechtl, H. F. R.; Beintema, D. J.: The neurological examination of the full-term newborn infant. Clinics in developmental medicine, No. 12 (Spastics International Medical Publications / Heinemann, London 1964).

Rutter, M.: Early sources of security and competence; in Bruner, Garton, Human growth and development (Clarendon Press, Oxford 1978).

Sameroff, A. J.; Chandler, M. J.: Reproductive risk and the continuum of caretaking casualty; in Horowitz, Hetherington, Scarr-Salapatek, Siegel, Review of child developmental research, vol. 4 (University of Chicago Press, Chicago 1975).

Seligman, M. E. P.: Helplessness. On depression, development and death (Freeman, San Francisco 1975).

Tinbergen, N.; Tinbergen, E. A.: Early childhood autism – an ethological approach. Z. Tierpsychol. *10:* 1–53 (1972).

Touwen, B. C. L.: Neurological development in infancy. Clinics in developmental medicine, No. 58 (Spastics International Medical Publications / Heinemann Medical Books, London 1976).

Trevarthen, C.: Conversations with a 2 month old. New Scient. *62:* 230–235 (1974).

Vlaar, H.; Alberts, E.: Adaptief, taktiel gedrag van moeders in de beginfase van de borstvoeding (Mother's adaptive tactile behaviour in the early phase of breastfeeding). Internal report, Laboratory of Experimental Clinical Psychology, Groningen 1980).

Watson, J. S.: Depression and the perception of control in early childhood; in Schulterbrandt, Raskin, Depression in childhood: diagnosis, treatment and conceptual models (Raven Press, New York 1977).

Werner, E. E.; Bierman, J. M.; French, F. E.: The children of Kauai (University of Hawaii, Honolulu 1977).

Prof. A. F. Kalverboer, PhD, Laboratory for Experimental Clinical Psychology, Turfsingel 46, NL-9712 KR Groningen (The Netherlands)

Adv. biol. Psychiat., vol. 11, pp. 95–113 (Karger, Basel 1983)

Periodicity in 'Schizophrenia'

Leiv R. Gjessing

Institute of Psychiatry, University of Bergen, Norway

Whereas periodicity of clinical syndromes is characteristic for manic-depressive disorders, it is rare within the 'schizophrenic' syndromes. It occurs especially in the catatonic patient, but the frequency of periodic catatonia is only about 2–3 % of all cases of dementia praecox.

Periodic catatonia was first mentioned by *Kirn* [12] in 1878, later by *Pilcz* [7], *Petrén* [6] and *Urstein* [11]. The syndrome was first described by *Kraepelin* [13] in 1913. It is characterized by periodically reappearing regular phases of catatonic excitement separated by regular intervals. The first description of periodic stupor was given by *Gjessing* [3] in 1932. The stupor cases are, however, very rare compared to the excitement cases.

This syndrome of periodic catatonia usually appears first after the patient has had several outbreaks of short duration or for many years has shown a 'schizophrenic' syndrome with catatonic, paranoid and/or hallucinatory features.

The periodic syndrome can last for years or disappears spontaneously, especially in younger people with short duration of illness. The duration of the periods varies from patient to patient, from days to weeks or months, but is quite regular for each patient.

In some cases the periodic excitement or stupor begins suddenly and both are very pronounced (synchronous syntonic type), whereas other irregular cases develop slowly and irregularly over several days with less-pronounced excitement and stupor (dys- or asynchronous syntonic types).

Table I. The effects of stimulation of the ergotropic and the trophotropic system

Stimulation of the posterior hypothalamus (ergotropic system)	Stimulation of the anterior hypothalamus (trophotropic system)
Autonomic effects	
Increased cardiac rate, blood pressure and sweat secretion	Reduction of cardiac rate, blood pressure and sweat secretion
Pupilary dilation	Pupilary constriction
Inhibited gastrointestinal, motor and secretory function	Increased gastrointestinal, motor and secretory function
Somatic effects	
Desynchrony of EEG	Synchrony of EEG
Increased skeletal muscle tone	Loss of skeletal muscle tone
Elevation of adrenaline, noradrenaline, thyroxine, adrenocortical steroids	Blocking of shivering response, increased secretion of insulin
Behavioral effects	
Arousal	Inactivity
Hightened activity and emotional responsiveness	Drowsiness
	Sleep

Clinical Features

By close observations of periodic catatonic patients, it is easy to discover changes in speech and behavior, in motor activity, and in functional activity of the vegetative nervous system.

Each patient has typical signs with peculiarities in speech and behavior a few hours to a few days before the onset of stupor or excitement. Just before stupor, the patients are more exited and restless, whereas patients going into excitement are more seclusive and taciturn. After stupor there is a certain degree of euphoria and after excitement inhibition and low spirits.

During the transition from the interval into the psychotic phase, the patient shows vegetative lability with a frequently changing pulse rate even in the course of the same day (50–110), and varying width of the pupil from hour to hour in spite of the same strength of light.

In the interval the amplitude of the temperature is usually reduced, falling within the lower normal range, whereas the pulse is between 60 and 80. In the psychotic phase temperature rises to 38°C and the pulse up to above 100.

During the interval and stupor or excitement, the trophotropic and the ergotropic vegetative nervous systems are stimulated cholinergically and adrenergically, respectively. *Gellhorn and Kiely* [1] have studied the stimulation of the posterior hypothalamus (ergotropic system) and the anterior hypothalamus (trophotropic system), as shown in table I.

All these autonomic, somatic and behaviorial effects of stimulations of the posterior and anterior hypothalamus are present in the psychotic and interval phase, respectively.

Clinical Course

The clinical course of regular periodic stupor (patient A_1) is presented in figure 1. The baseline separates the degree of stupor below the line from the degree of alertness above the line, measured as the ability to consentrate. After dental extraction in November 1927 (b) and controlled diet since November 1928 (c) the periods were very regular until they disappeared after thyroxine treatment in April 1929. In January 1935 he relapsed on the fifth day after operation for a suppurative perforated appendix. After two stupor phases he was again treated successfully with thyroxine. In April 1940 he had his last relapse following insufficient thyroid medication, but recovered after thyroxine. After that he was in good health and working until he died aged 82 years in 1978.

Regular periodic exitement (patient B_1) is illustrated in figure 2. This patient had 17 phases of psychomotor excitement with depressive intervals and since thyroxine treatment in 1934 no relapse.

Periodic psychomotor excitement (patient C_2) over a period of 10 years is shown in figure 3. After he was put on a H diet, containing only milk, cream, sugar, 2 eggs, 2 g NaCl, water and vitamins in January 1935, the interval was prolonged by almost 5 months, and the following excited phases were less severe. After thyroxine was given in March 1936 he recovered but had two relapses due to insufficient thyroid medication.

The 3 above-mentioned cases were all treated with thyroxine and dry thyroid substance. Another patient (B_2) with periodic excitement, however, recovered spontaneously (fig. 4). The course was irregular during the first few months. From March 1940, he was given a standardized H-diet and regular periods of excitement appeared. After about 1 year with regular periods of excitement, they suddenly disappeared and the patient recovered completely during the following 12 months.

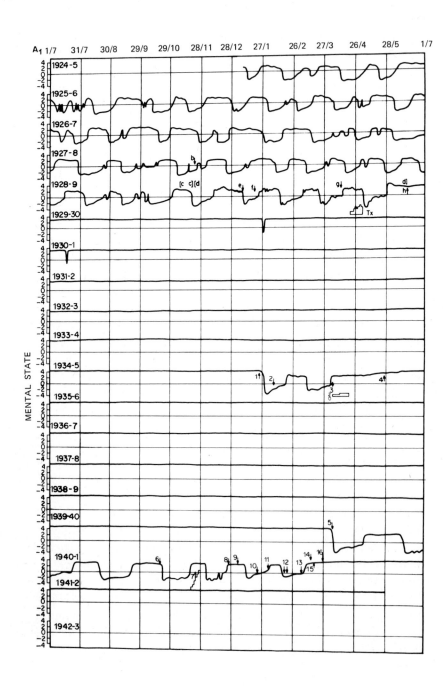

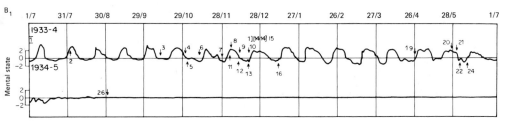

Fig. 2. Patient B_1. Admitted to Dikemark 2/6/33. The diagram shows his phases of psychomotor excitement. The periodicity was already fully established on admission. It was controlled from June 1934 onwards after the administration of 41 mg thyroxine (25/4–6/5/34).

In order to illustrate the course of irregular catatonic phases the record of patient H. K. is shown in figure 5. Here, phases of catatonic excitement during approximately 18 months occurs more or less regularly or irregularly, probably because of thyroxine intervention in a patient who lacked all drive and insight.

Another example of irregular catatonia without periodicity is shown in figure 6. After removal of chronic infection (fig. 6, 2 and 3) he was given thyroxine and thyroid tablets without any effect (fig. 6, 7 and 8).

In some cases the seasons seem to influence the occurrence of catatonic phases. In figure 7 it is easy to see how the catatonic attacks in patient C_1 are present with a maximum intensity in the middle of the winter. In addition, the N-balance shows a seasonal periodicity similar to that of the air temperature. From January 1940, these two curves, however, run opposite

---

Fig. 1. The clinical course of patient A_1. The baseline (0) separates the degree of stupor below the line from the degree of alertness above the line, measured as the ability to concentrate. Metabolic studies were made from March to June 1925, November 1928–June 1929. In May 1929, his disturbances were controlled by thyroid medication. (Tx indicates in steps 3, 4, 5, 4, 5, 6, and 5 mg thyroxine daily in 1929 which was followed by dried thyroid extract.) January 30 he relapsed for 3 days following insufficient thyroid administration and relapsed again in July 1930 after a too high intake of protein and nucleic acid. August 1930–January 1935 he was symptom free. However, on the fifth day after operation for a suppurative perforated appendix he again relapsed. After two stupor phases he was again successfully treated with thyroxine, 2 mg daily followed by 3 mg daily, followed by dried thyroid extract. April 1940 he had his last relapse, following insufficient thyroid medication. This time, medication was given out of phase with the nitrogen retention and it took three periods of stupor before the symptoms were controlled. Letters and figures in diagram indicate: b 1927 = 23/11 dental extraction; c 1928 = 9–23/11 on controlled diet; d = 24/11/ 28–13/6/29 H diet:1,500 ml milk, 200 ml cream, 50 g sugar, 3 eggs, 2.5 g Bemax [fig. 1–14 from ref. 4].

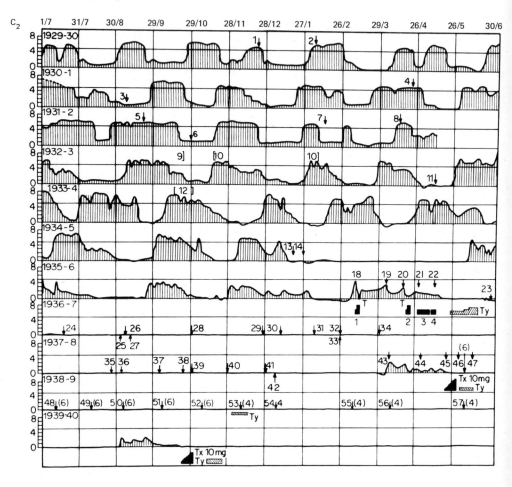

Fig. 3. Patient C_2. Diagram showing phases of psychomotor excitement, 1/7/29–30/6/40. Note the interval from 15/1 to 9/6/35 (almost 5 months), after he was put on H-diet on 15/1; and the two relapses after 22 and 15 months, respectively (insufficient hormone therapy), on each of which occasions we intervened with thyroxine and dry thyroid.

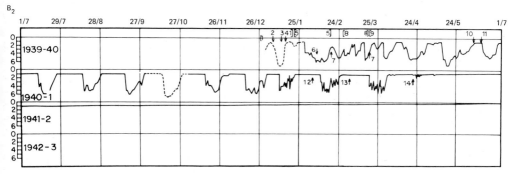

Fig. 4. Patient B₂. Diagram showing phases of catatonic excitement. 0 = No defect of concentration; 6 = maximal impairment. Irregular course during the first few months. From 20/3/40 onwards, standardized H diet and regular periods. From 15/1/41, metabolism recorded. Recovered spontaneously.

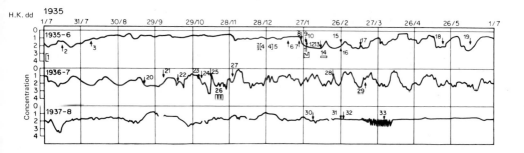

Fig. 5. Patient H.K. Diagram covering period 1/7/35–1/7/38, showing fall in patient's powers of concentration: 0 = normal, 4 = maximum impairment (bordering on stupor). Patient admitted to Dikemark 27/6/35. After 2 months he was relatively rational, fully orientated, behaved well, but lacked all drive and insight. Even course till the end of January 1936. From then on (probably because of thyroxine intervention: 3 mg daily from 10 to 15/2/35) there followed 18 months of catatonic excited phases which occurred sometimes irregularly and sometimes more regularly (May–September 1936; March–June 1937); thereafter, the course of the illness is again more even, though concentration is at a much reduced level.

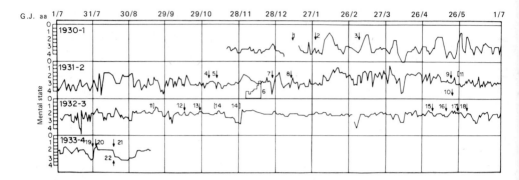

Fig. 6. This mental state of this patient varied with some periodicity to begin with after dental treatment (2) and tonsillectomy (3), but later the course was irregular without any periodicity. No effect of thyoxine (6) or thyroid tablets. This patient suddenly got depressed for no good reason in 1929, 26 years old. After a few weeks he was preoccupied and apathetic, lacking all spontaneity in a twilight state, with ideas of persecution and catatonic features.

to each other as a sign of spontaneous decrease of the protein deposit in the organism. The patient was only treated with the H-diet (milk, cream, eggs, water, salts and vitamins).

The clinical course seems to be influenced by acute and chronic infection (case A_1), by H-diet (cases A_1, C_2, B_2 and C_1), by season (C_1), and most markedly by thyroxine and dried thyroid substance (A_1, B_1, C_2 and H. K.?).

The effect of successful intervention with thyroxine and dry thyroid in patient A_1, B_1 and C_2 is clearly shown in figure 8.

The low ability to mental concentrations is normalized and the low O_2 consumption in the interval is elevated.

Single Period

In order to illustrate the interval, the switch into the psychotic phase and the psychotic phase itself, the pulse and temperature recording in patients A_1, B_2 and C_1 is useful (fig. 9, 10). The psychotic phase is usually heralded days in advance by changes in pulse and body temperature (except for C_1 10/4/37).

By looking more closely into the other somatic parameters in patient A_1 in figure 11, the motor activity, which is determined seismographically,

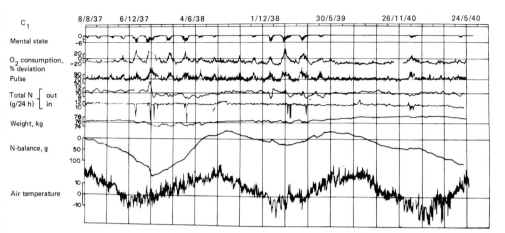

Fig. 7. Patient C_1. Influence of the seasons, 8/8/37–7/4/40. Admitted to Dikemark 23/1/37 after 20 years of illness. From 3/4/37 on H-diet. Regular periodicity in summer and autumn 1937, though with only very mild phases of excitement. Winter (December 1937 to May 1938) as before. Summer 1938, completely free from attack for 2 months. December 1938 to May 1939, only 3 severe phases of excitement. Thereafter, phases completely under control from mid-May to the end of December, when there was again a mild reaction phase. March 1940, slightly ill-tempered for 2 days. The pre-1937 picture, with irregular periodicity and severe excitement at all seasons, i.e. with no apparent seasonal influence, gradually disappears with the introduction of H-diet and controlled metabolic routine, as the patient's regulatory capacity clearly improves. To begin with it was only in summer that the patient could regulate against functional disturbances, but after he improved he could do this in winter as well. The critical change from insufficiency to sufficiency came in January 1940. While the N-balance shows a seasonal periodicity rather similar to that of the air temperature (minimal N-balance occurring 1–2 months after minimal temperature), from January 1940 the curves for N-balance and for air temperature run opposite to each other: the protein deposit in the organism decreases spontaneously, and in the same way as in other cases was achieved only by means of thyroxine therapy.

illustrates very well the prestupor excitation and the sudden fall to akinesia at the onset of the stupor. Otherwise oxygen consumption is synchronous with pulse rate, hemoglobin and nitrogen in blood, whereas erythrocyte sedimentation is 0–1 mm at the onset of stupor.

In figure 12 the N-excretion show phasic flucturations and the curves for titrable acids and NH_3 follow the same course. The degree of concordance in the course of the curves is striking.

This regular periodicity of somatic symptoms are even better illustrated in patient B_1 (fig. 13). Here the urinary excretion of N, titrable

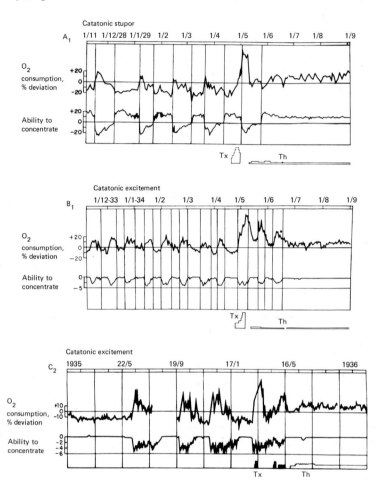

Fig. 8. Patients A_1, B_1, and C_2. Oxygen consumption and concentration during the spontaneous course of catatonic periods, during intervention with thyroxine and dry thyroid, and after successful intervention. Note how in the spontaneous course of the illness, the two curves (which were recorded independently) run opposite to each other; after intervention with thyroxine this relationship changes to a normal one of high oxygen consumption associated with high concentration.

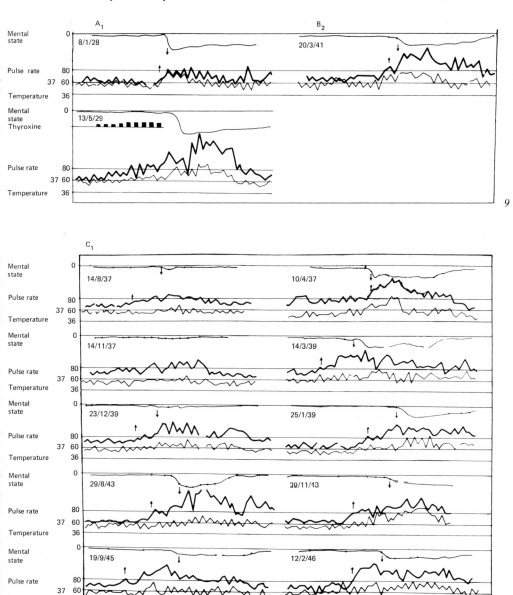

Fig. 9, 10. These figures show how the reaction phase is usually heralded days in advance by changes in pulse rate and body temperature (except for C_1, 10/4/37. ↓ = First day of reaction phase; ↑ = first sign of rise in pulse and temperature; A_1: black rectangles = thyroxine.

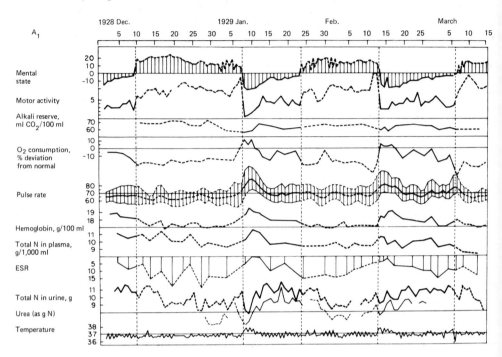

Fig. 11. Patient A_1. Two catatonic periods, 10/12/28–24/1/29 and 24/1–7/3/29, each covering an interval phase, in which the patient is awake, and the succeeding phase of stupor. Mental state is given in rough schematic form in the top line. Motor activity: determined seismographically. Note the prestupor (like prenarcotic) excitation, and the sudden fall to akinesia at onset of stupor. The alkali reserve shows slight acidosis, well ahead o onset of stupor. Note the fall in BMR (O_2 consumption) in the interval, in spite of the increase in movement, and the sudden rise at onset of stupor, in spite of total akinesia. The BMR curve is synchronous and syntonic with those showing pulse rate, hemoglobin, and nitrogen in blood (increased concentration at onset of stupor). ESR increases in the interval, 0–1 mm at onset of stupor. Total N and urea excretion are low in the interval, rising shortly after the onset of stupor. *Temperature* rises on the first few days of stupor.

acidity, NH_3-N, urine pH, NaCl and daily urine volume are determined during day and night separately during two periods, each lasting 23 days, but separated by 43 days.

These recordings yield astonishingly similar results as there is very little difference between the corresponding days of the two periods. This fact provides evidence that the underlying processes form a chain reaction which unfolds in a very regular pattern, and indicates that the periodicity is

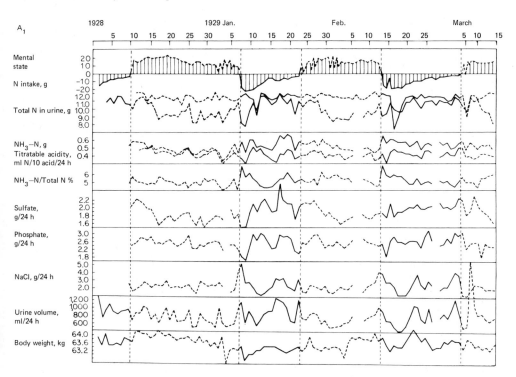

Fig. 12. Patient A_1. Mental state, N intake, total N in urine, NH_3, titratable acidity, NH_3 % of total nitrogen, sulfate, phosphate, NaCl, daily urine volume, and body weight in the same two catatonic periods as figure 12. Note the refusal of food (vomiting) at the beginning of each stupor phase. Total N excretion shows phasic fluctuations. The curves for titratable acids and NH_3 follow the same course. The degree of concordance in the couse of the curves is striking, particularly shortly before and after each onset of stupor; compare the steep rise in NH_3 and of the excretion of NaCl and of urine, before the stupor.

not governed by exogenous complications but is spontaneous and purely endogenous.

Figure 14 which covers 10 months of patient B_1, illustrates both the periodicity of all the different functions recorded and how these fluctuations gradually disappear after intervention with thyroxine and thyroid extract.

The catecholamines and sleep are also studied in another patient (fig. 15). Here the pulse rate, the BMR and norepinephrine and epinephrine are corresponding to each other and all are elevated during the stupor phase. The sleep parameters, the actual sleep time and the REM

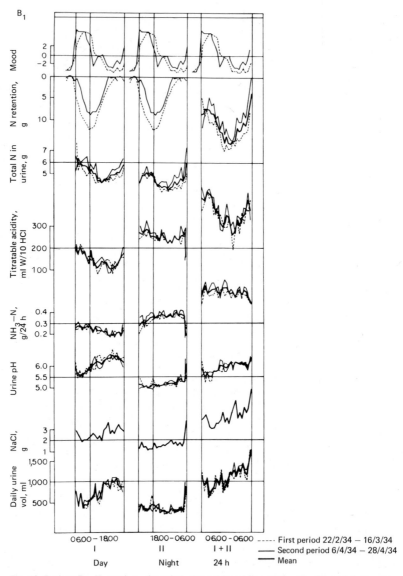

Fig. 13. Patient B₁. Excretion of total N, titratable acidity, NH₃–N, pH, and daily urine volume divided into day-time excretion (06.00–18.00) and night-time (18.00–06.00) for days 1–23 in two periods (22/2–16/3/34 and 6/4–28/4/34). The thick line is the mean of the two portions obtained on corresponding days of the two periods (i. e. 43 days apart: 2/2 and 6/4/34; 23/2 and 7/4/34; and so on). The right-hand column shows the summation of 24-hour portions and their mean values. Although the corresponding tests are 43 days apart, there is very little difference between them, which probably points to a chain reaction process.

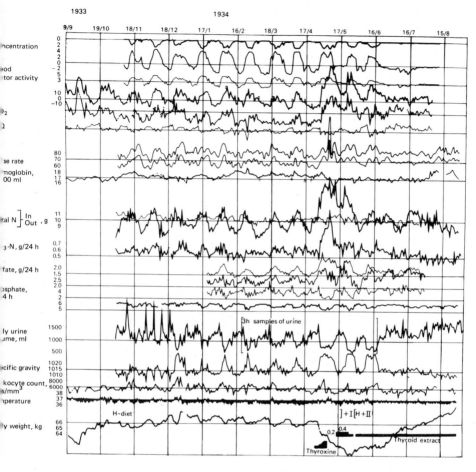

Fig. 14. Patient D_1. This figure, which covers about 10 months, shows the periodicity found in all functions recorded, especially O_2 consumption, total N excretion, and daily urine volume. Note also how the fluctuations disappear after intervention with thyroxine and thyroid extract, especially O_2 consumption, pulse, and daily urine volume. (The period in question does not cover the deterioration in the curve for total N excretion.)

time, are both markedly reduced during the stupor phase and is slightly elevated in the end of the interval.

When this patient is treated with reserpin (fig. 16), the psychotic phases disappear, the BMR drops to low levels, the norepinephrine, epinephrine and their metabolites decrease, but dopamine and its acidic metabolite are not reduced. Disulfiram has a similar effect (fig. 16).

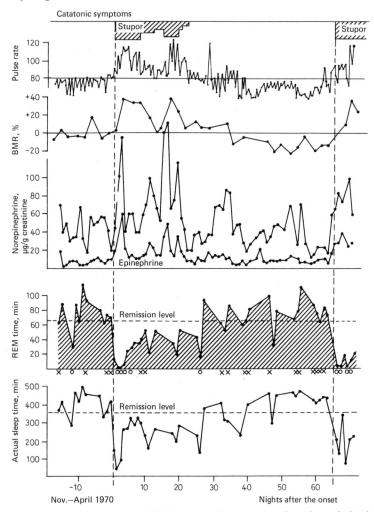

Fig. 15. Longitudinal study of EEG sleep and urinary excretion of catecholamines, as well as pulse rate and BMR, in relation to clinical state throughout the transition phase to active phase and further to the next active phase is shown. The abscissa represents the number of days or nights after the onset of catatonic symptoms. The levels of epinephrine and norepinephrine in 24-hour specimens each day are charted on the middle graphs. REM time and actual sleep time measures are recorded on the two lowest graphs. The mean values of sleep time levels in the remission phase of the patient are indicated by the dashed horizontal lines. REM time, as well as actual sleep time, abruptly fell to the bottom immediately after the onset of stupor, together with huge amounts of urinary epinephrine and norepinephrine excretion. 66 days after the onset, the same pattern was observed. Circles under the baseline of REM time graph indicate the REM latency prolonged more than 180 min, and crosses indicate the REM latency shortened less than 30 min [from ref. 10].

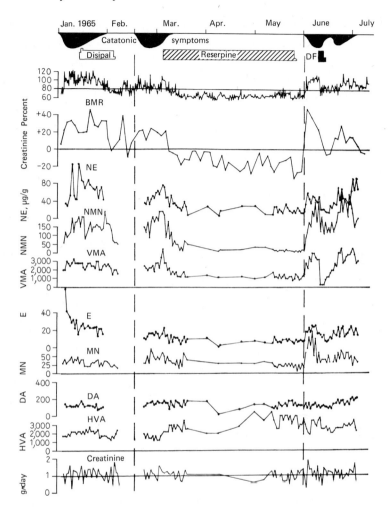

Fig. 16. Effect of reserpine and disulfiram on catatonic state and the urinary excretion of catecholamines and their metabolites. Graphs in this figure are shown in the same way as figure 2. The drugs administered during this period were Disipal: orphenadrine-HCl 200 mg, reserpine 3 mg and DF: disulfiram 1.2 g a day [from ref. 10].

Pathogenesis in Catatonia

All these figures show how the periods can be very regular, especially after removal of acute or chronic infection and on a standardized diet. The periodicity can be counteracted or suppressed by thyroxine and dry thyroid treatment or even easier by psychotropic drugs like α-methyldopa, reserpine, disulfiram, haloperidol or chlorpromazin, which interfere with the catecholamine metabolism. These facts bring both the thyroid gland and the catecholamine metabolism into the pathogenesis of the periodicity.

Thyroxine, however, only works on regular periodic cases, not on dys- or asynchronous cases. But how does it work? Is the thyroid gland insufficient since thyroxine treatment elevates metabolism? Or does thyroxine stimulate specific enzymes (peptidases?) which inactivates psychotic metabolites (peptides?) in the brain? What about the antipsychotic drugs? Do they interfere with the synthesis or breakdown of certain psychotic metabolites (peptides?)?

Richter [8] emphazises that in nearly all instances of periodic diseases 'the simultaneous existence of two phenomena must be considered: a basic illness and a periodic mechanism. Our study has revealed the existence of a definite relationship between those two phenomena in that periodicity when it exists, recurrently in one phase exaggerates, then in the other phase reduces or eliminates the symptoms that were originally present – but does not bring out new symptoms.'

It is possible that thyroxine mainly removes the periodicity, and that by eliminating the psychotic periods the patient recovers.

The antipsychotic drugs, however, may act on psychotic metabolites causing psychotic symptoms independent of periodicity. But again by eliminating the psychotic symptoms, the patient recovers.

The strict periodicity of the regular periodic catatonia points to an accumulation of some active metabolites which may be produced centrally during the interval. Reaching a certain level, this hypothetic active compound (peptide?) may act as a strong stimulus to the noradrenergic nervous system and precipitate the psychotic signs and symptoms. In nonperiodic catatonia, other metabolites may be in operation since thyroxine is not effective. Antipsychotic drugs, however, are active against the psychotic symptoms, but the patient may not recover completely.

Further studies of active peptides in the cerebrospinal fluid and in brain biopsy may, however, give more insight into the pathogenesis of catatonia.

Summary

Periodicity in 'schizophrenia' is rare and mainly present in catatonia. In some cases, the periodic stupor or excitement occurs suddenly, regularly and pronounced (synchroneous types). In other cases, the psychotic phases start more slowly and are more irregular and less pronounced (dys- or asynchronic). The clinical features and the clinical course of periodic catatonic patients as well s the single period are illustrated in order to discuss the pathogenesis. Periodic catatonia seems to be due to a basic illnes ('schizophrenia') as well as to a dysregulation causing periodicity. The strict periodicity indicates an accumulation of an active psychosis-promoting metabolite (peptide?).

References

1   Gellhorn, E.; Kiely, F.: The physiology and pharmacology of sleep; in Mendels, Biological psychiatry (Wiley, New York 1973).
2   Gjessing, R.: Beiträge zur Kenntnis der Pathophysiologie des katatonen Stupors. I. Über periodisch rezidivierenden katatonen Stupor, mit kritischem Beginn und Abschluss. Arch. Psychiat. NervKrank. *96:* 319–392 (1932).
3   Gjessing, R.: Beiträge zur Kenntnis der Pathophysiologie des katatonen Stupors. II. Über aperiodisch rezidivierend verlaufenden katatonen Stupor, mit lytischem Beginn und Abschluss. Arch. Psychiat. NervKrank. *96:* 393–473 (1933).
4   Gjessing, R.: Contribution to the somatology of periodic catatonia (Pergamon Press, Oxford 1976).
5   Kraepelin, E.: Psychiatrie. Ein Lehrbuch für Studierende und Ärzte (Barth, Leipzig 1909).
6   Petrén, A.: Über Spätheilungen von Psychosen (Nordstedt, Stockholm 1908).
7   Pilcz, A.: Die periodischen Geistesstörungen. Lehrbuch der speziellen Psychiatrie (Fischer, Jena 1901).
8   Richter, C. P.: Biological clocks in medicine and psychiatry (Thomas, Springfield 1965).
9   Takahashi, S.; Gjessing, L. R.: Periodic catatonia. III. Longitudinal sleep study with urinary excretion of catecholamines. J. psychiat. Res. *9:* 123–139 (1972).
10 Takahashi, S.; Gjessing, L. R.: Studies of periodic catatonia. IV. Longitudinal study of catecholamine metabolism, with and without drugs. J. psychiat. Res. *9:* 293–314 (1972).
11 Urstein, J.: Die Dementia praecox (Urban & Schwarzenberg, Berlin 1909).
12 Kirn (1878).
13 Kraeplin (1913).

L. R. Gjessing, MD, Institute of Psychiatry, University of Bergen, Helleveien 65, N-5000 Bergen (Norway)

Adv. biol. Psychiat., vol. 11, pp. 114–127 (Karger, Basel 1983)

Circadian Rhythms in Affective Disorders

Body Temperature and Sleep Physiology in Endogenous Depressives

Domien G. M. Beersma, Rudi H. van den Hoofdakker,
Hans W. B. M. van Berkestijn[1]

Department of Biological Psychiatry, Psychiatric University Clinic, Groningen,
The Netherlands

Introduction

In the last few years, two types of imperfections in rhythms have been suggested as causes of endogenous depression. Oral temperature data for manic depressives were interpreted by *Kripke* et al. [1978] as showing desynchronization of the temperature rhythm with respect to the 24-hour periodicity in the natural environment and, thus, with respect to the entrained 24-hour sleep-wake cycle. According to their hypothesis, the magnitude of the time lag between temperature oscillation and environmental rhythmicity would, in some way, be of importance to the patient's mood. *Wehr and Wirz-Justice* [1981] collected data from studies in the literature in which measurements were carried out on biological rhythms in depressives and controls. They concluded, from differences in acrophase times of a series of such rhythms, that there would be a phase advance of some of these rhythms in depression. The evidence for a relative phase advance of the rapid eye movement (REM) sleep and body temperature cycles with respect to the sleep-wake cycle was especially emphasized by them. This evidence is based on the frequently observed short REM sleep latencies, long first REM sleep episodes, and large duration of REM sleep in the first third of the night [*Wehr and Wirz-Justice,* 1981]. These phenomena are interpreted as a shift in the circadian REM sleep production such that its maximum occurs in the first instead of the last part of sleep.

[1] We thank Dr. *A. L. Bouhuys* for many inspiring discussions. We are further grateful to Mr. *W. Stadman* for drawing the figures, to Mr. *C. Tauber* for correcting and to Mrs. *M. Alkema* for typing the manuscript.

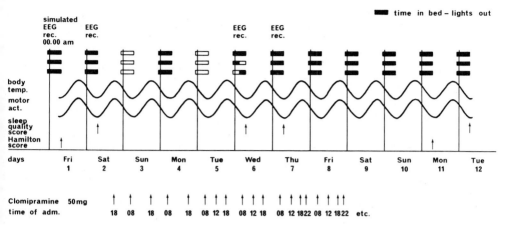

Fig. 1. Design. Explanation: see text.

Some data would also indicate a forward shift of the maxima and minima of body temperature [*Cahn* et al., 1968; *Atkinson* et al., 1975].

In a study currently in progress, we are measuring core body temperature and motor activity continously during a period of 11 days and we are making sleep recordings during a number of nights in endogenous depressives. The study is aimed primarily at improving a biological therapy, which is based on antidepressant medication in combination with a strictly controlled sleep-wake schedule. In the present paper, the data obtained in this study will be used to test the above-mentioned hypotheses.

Design

Subjects were 27 inpatients (15 women, mean age 51 ± ‹SD› 13 years; range 22–69 years) of the Department of Biological Psychiatry, of the University Hospital, Groningen, the Netherlands. The diagnosis of endogenous depression was confirmed by either of two psychiatrists (*R.v.d.H., H.v.B.*). The mean score on the Hamilton Rating Scale [*Hamilton*, 1967] was 32 ± 5. Important aspects of the design, which was based on results obtained in previous studies [*Elsenga and van den Hoofdakker*, 1980; *van Bemmel and van den Hoofdakker*, 1981], are summarized in figure 1. Three groups of patients are treated with clomipramine and two sleep deprivations. One group is allowed 3 h of sleep during the first half of the second recovery night, the second group 3 h during the last half of that night; the third group is permitted ad libitum sleep. During the 11-day experimental period, rectal temperature and motor activity of the nondominant arm are continuously recorded using a Medilog cassette recorder.

Standard sleep recordings [*Rechtschaffen and Kales,* 1968] are made during the nights after days 1, 5, and 6. During the night before day 1, electrodes were attached to adapt the patients to equipment and procedure. The Hamilton Rating Scale for depression was completed on days 1 and 11. A sleep quality rating scale [*Mulder-Hajonides van der Meulen* et al., 1980] was completed early in the mornings of days 2, 5, 7, and 12. The scheme of the administration of clomipramine is also presented in figure 1. All patients gave informed consent and were free of psychopharmacological medication for at least 3.5 days before the beginning of the experimental period. For the analysis of the sleep data, we used the polygrams of the baseline nights in all 27 patients. However, because of 6 dropouts and technical failures in 6 other cases, we are, at present, able to analyze temperature and activity data for only 15 patients.

Results

Core Body Temperature

Temperature curves during the first 36 h (roughly the time span between the start of the measurements and the first administration of drugs, see fig. 1) are of good quality in 11 patients. These are presented in figure 2. It is evident from these registrations that temperature is high during both days and low during the intervening night. 3 of the 11 patients are classified as bipolar depressives. Temperature curves of these patients are presented at the top of figure 2. The curves do not deviate clearly from the other curves. We will, therefore, make no further differentiation between these types of depressives. We find no obvious phase differences between individual curves. This result would be highly improbable if desynchronization of the temperature rhythm were the general cause of depressed mood in our patients. In that case, a randomly distributed series of phase positions would be expected. Signs of phase advance of the temperature rhythms are also not obviously present.

These conclusions, however, are justified only when the temperature curve is considered as reflecting some endogenous biological rhythm, i. e., a

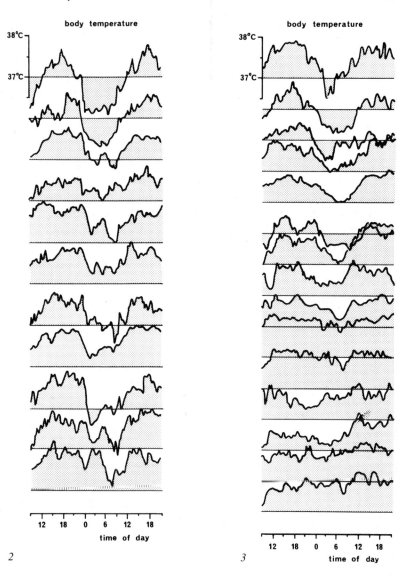

Fig. 2. The course of body temperature over 36 h in 11 medication-free patients. Sleep was permitted.

Fig. 3. The course of body temperature over 36 h without sleep in 15 patients. Each curve presents the mean of two 36-hour periods (see fig. 1).

rhythm which is neither generated nor triggered by external influences. It is known that the sleep-wake schedule clearly influences rectal temperature, as is demonstrated, for example, in sleep deprivation studies [Åkerstedt et al., 1979; *Wever,* 1979]. However, since this masking phenomenon is strictly coupled to the sleep-wake rhythm, it cannot be part of an endogenous rhythm of body temperature. As a consequence, desynchronization of the endogenous temperature rhythm could be masked by sleep. If this is the case, the nocturnal part of the temperature curve would always show the lowest temperature values, irrespective of the phase position of some endogenous oscillation. Hence, studying temperature under normal sleep-wake conditions is not in and of itself adequate to prove or disprove either desynchronization or phase advance. A better strategy is to analyze temperature curves obtained under conditions where the masking effect of sleep is absent, i. e., during sleep deprivation.

Temperature curves of the days during which sleep deprivation was carried out (days 2 and 4) are available for 15 patients. The averages over the 2 days are plotted in figure 3. The curves are more or less arranged in sequence of decreasing amplitudes. Only the 8 upper curves show sufficient modulation to determine the approximate locations of extreme values. As in the curves obtained under normal sleep conditions (fig. 2), no rhythm disturbances are apparent in these 8 curves. The circadian modulation in the remaining 7 curves at the bottom of figure 3 is almost zero. This set of flat curves, of course, does not allow any conclusion with regard to phase positions.

Hence, *none of the curves show desynchronization of the body temperature rhythm,* irrespective of whether sleep was permitted. On the other hand, the phase advance hypothesis is not easily tested with these data because measurements performed under identical conditions in healthy subjects are not available. Further, we did not obtain comparable data from the same patients during remission. Nevertheless, the troughs in the temperature curves (when present) seem to occur at normal times of day and, therefore, large phase advances of the temperature rhythm are unlikely.

Apart from the fact that the 7 above-mentioned curves without clear circadian modulation do not contribute to the test of either the desynchronization or the phase advance hypothesis, they deserve more extensive discussion. Apparently, some subjects do not show any rhythmicity in body temperature at all when they are deprived of sleep. Their sleep-wake alternations seem to completely control the highs and lows in body

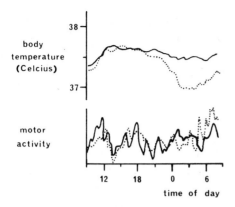

Fig. 4. Body temperature and motor activity over 24 h without sleep. Solid lines = Mean curves of patients without clear circadian modulation in body temperature; dotted lines = patients with circadian modulation in body temperature.

temperature. A possible explanation of this lack of modulation might be a masking influence of increased motor activity during the period in which sleep would otherwise have taken place. As mentioned above, we measured motor activity of the nondominant arm in all patients. In figure 4, the means of the curves with and without clear circadian modulation in temperature are shown together with the means of the motor activity curves. The similarity of the distribution of motor activity over the days in both subgroups is rather large. Therefore, it is not likely that a difference in motor activity is the cause of the flattening of the temperature curve in some depressed patients. So, in some patients the sleep-wake alternations seem to determine completely the highs and lows in body temperature. In the many rhythm studies with healthy subjects [*Wever, 1979*], this phenomenon has never been reported. In the experiments described in the literature, a sleep-wake rhythm with a period beyond the range of 23–27 h was never synchronized with the temperature rhythm. This finding can only be explained if one assumes that the endogenous modulation in the temperature rhythm of healthy subjects has a higher amplitude than the masking effect of sleep. This experimental result in a large healthy population thus contrasts considerably with our findings in 7 of 15 depressives.

At this point it seems possible to classify our population of depressed patients on the basis of physiological data. Some patients show little or no temperature modulation, while others seem to show quite normal amplitudes of temperature oscillations. Although the population is rela-

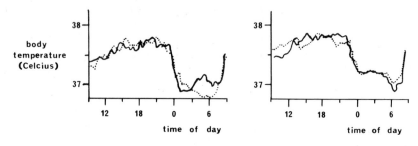

Fig. 5. Temperature curves on day 1 (solid lines) and day 11 (dotted lines). *a* Means for 4 patients who improved considerably. *b* 4 patients who did not improve.

tively small, it is still interesting to see whether the subdivision suggested might be related to other characteristics. However, both subgroups contain males as well as females, young as well as elderly patients, and bipolar as well as unipolar depressives. Furthermore, we found no indication of a relationship between the amplitude of the temperature rhythm and the severity of the depression at the start of the experiment, nor did we find the amplitude to be of predictive value for improvement. Apparently, the phenomenon of constant temperature during days including sleep deprivation is not strongly connected to any of these other variables. However, the phenomenon seems to be patient dependent. Whenever one sleep deprivation day shows a flat temperature curve, so does the other.

The available data permit another way of testing the validity of the phase advance hypothesis. Temperature was measured over a period of 11 days. On the average, patients improved, as indicated by a decline of the Hamilton scores between days 1 and 11. We selected the 4 patients with the greatest improvement (17, 18, 28, and 29 Hamilton units, respectively) and the 4 patients showing the least improvement (1, 4, 7, and 7 Hamilton units, respectively). The mean temperature curves of these groups on both the baseline day 1 and day 11 of the experiment are presented in figure 5a, b. Again, it is obvious from the curves that there is no major circadian component showing a phase advance in the presence of depression. The only difference which might be of significance is the shift, upon improvement in the clinical state, of the temperature minimum to the later part of the night (fig. 5a). Whether or not these differences in nocturnal temperature curves are significant should be determined in a much larger population of patients observed during depression and remission. It must be remarked, however, that such differences in body temperature are quite

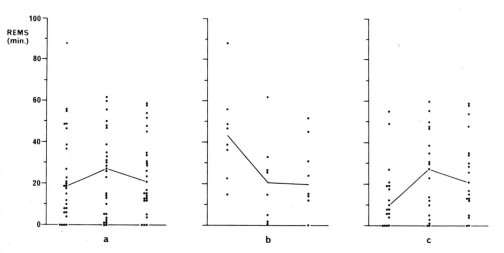

Fig. 6. REM sleep duration per third of the sleep period. *a* Data for 27 depressives. *b* 8 nights are selected in which REM sleep occurred within 10 min after sleep onset. *c* The remaining 19 nights.

probably related to a difference in sleep quality. Examination of the sleep quality scores has lead to results in accordance with this view. The subgroup of patients who improved most started with severe complaints regarding the first night of sleep, whereas they considered their last night to be of very high quality. Additional evidence in favor of the influence of sleep quality on temperature stems from observations in the subgroup of patients who improved the least. Here, the difference in shape of the temperature curves is very small, if it is present at all. According to their scores, these patients suffered from equally bad sleep quality during both nights.

Finally some remarks must be made on the possibility of the influence of the antidepressant drug. The temperature curves used in our argument were obtained after drug treatment started. It might therefore be possible that the temperature curves are influenced in such a way that phase abnormalities have disappeared or that circadian modulation is decreased. Although it seems to be rather unlikely that all our conclusions are based on drug artifacts, similar experiments must be done under drugfree conditions.

Sleep Physiology

From a circadian point of view, sleep physiology is of interest because the REM sleep production has been reported to show circadian modulation [*Czeisler* et al., 1980]. As noted in the introduction, the maximum of the production of REM sleep is considered to be shifted forward in depressive patients. The most frequently mentioned parameters are short REM sleep latency and high REM sleep production in the first third of the sleep period. The short mean REM sleep latency is well documented [*Kupfer and Foster*, 1972; *Schulz* et al., 1979]. It is noteworthy that REM sleep latencies show a bimodal distribution, i. e., REM sleep appears either very early or after a normal time span. The phenomenon of sleep onset REM sleep periods (SOREMPS) is also found in the baseline sleep of 8 out of our 27 patients. The apparent existence of two very distinct classes of REM sleep latency values suggests strongly that the two subgroups should be compared with respect to other physiological characteristics.

First, we shall consider the distribution of REM sleep over the night. In figure 6a, the median values for the time spent in REM sleep per third of the sleep period are shown for the entire population of 27 EEG recordings.

Note: The sleep period usually is defined as extending from the first occurence of stage 2 until the last occurrence of stage 2. However, the EEG of depressed patients is characterized by an abundance of stage shifts. Sometimes the first occurrence of stage 2 is followed by 1 h of wakefulness. In such cases, the first 20-second epoch scored as stage 2 does not seem to define sleep onset. To overcome such difficulties we decided to define the sleep period as extending from the first sequence of 2 min of sleep (stages 2, 3, 4, or REM) until the last sequence of 2 min of sleep.

The curve presented closely resembles the results described in the literature. However, when we subdivide the data on the basis of short and normal REM sleep latencies (fig. 6b, c), a large difference in REM sleep production during the first third of the sleep period can be seen. During the first third of the sleep periods beginning with SOREMPs, about three times more REM sleep is produced than in the analogous portion of the sleep periods with normal REM sleep latencies. Thus, the well-known flat distribution presented in figure 6a is, in fact, the result of superimposition of two completely different distributions.

The sleep period usually consists of 4 or 5 ultradian cycles, each of which includes a certain amount of time spent in REM sleep. Subdivision of such a series of cycles into three equal fractions carries the risk of misinterpretation of the results by interference artifacts. In order to overcome such artifacts, we have chosen to study the distribution of REM sleep production by the use of plots of REM sleep accumulation over time. In figure 7a, this type of data presentation has been applied for both the

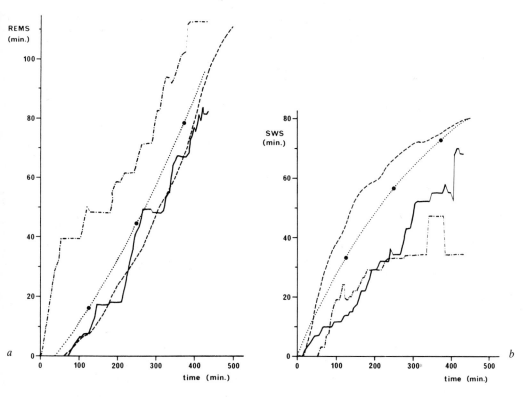

Fig. 7. REM sleep accumulation *(a)* and SWS accumulation *(b)*. Solid lines = Median accumulation in 19 nights in which REM sleep latency was more than 10 min; dashed and dotted lines = median accumulation in 8 nights in which REMS latency was less than 10 min; dashed lines = accumulation curves obtained by *Gaillard* [1977]; dotted lines = accumulation calculated on the basis of data from *Spiegel* [1981].

SOREMP sleep periods and the periods with normal REM sleep latencies. The dashed and dotted line shows the median REM sleep accumulation curve in minutes for the 8 SOREMP sleep periods; the continuous curve shows the 19 sleep periods with normal REM sleep latencies. It is obvious that the curves differ distinctly in the first hour of sleep. During this hour in the SOREMP nights, a total of more than 30 min of REM sleep was produced, whereas in the non-SOREMP nights no REM sleep was produced. Thereafter, the curves appear to run roughly in parallel, indicating that the per-hour production of REM sleep is about the same during SOREMP sleep and non-SOREMP sleep. Differences between these two sleep types are thus limited to the first hour after sleep onset.

Since the non-SOREMP sleep is characterized by normal REM sleep latencies, it is of interest to know to what extent the non-SOREMP REM sleep accumulation curve deviates from similar curves for healthy controls. A comparison is possible with data from *Gaillard and Martin* [1975]. These authors present a REM sleep accumulation curve obtained from 26 recordings in 13 young healthy men. Their curve is replotted in figure 7a. The similarity between *Gaillard and Martin's* [1975] data and our non-SOREMP data is striking. Another set of data suitable for comparison with our own is that of *Spiegel* [1981]. This author presents the number of minutes spent in REM sleep per third of the second EEG night in 57 elderly (55–70 years) individuals. From these data we calculated the median amount of time from sleep onset and the median amount of time spent in REM sleep. The dotted line in figure 7a represents the parabola through these three points. Apparently, the REM sleep accumulation of our endogenously depressed patients with normal REMS latency does not deviate from similar curves measured in elderly people.

This result indicates that the difference in the distribution of REM sleep production during the night between depressives and controls is very likely caused by a subgroup of sleep periods in depressives in which SOREMPS occur. These sleep periods differ only in the first hour of sleep from nights with normal REM sleep latencies. In our opinion, these results make it impossible to interpret the existing data on REM sleep production as evidence for a phase advance in depression. Our findings suggest the alternative interpretation that REM sleep production in depressives is quite normal, except for a sleep onset disturbance which occurs in 20–30 % of the nights.

Apart from abnormalities in REM sleep production also disturbances of slow wave sleep (SWS) production are reported in depressives [*Gillin* et al., 1979]. It is interesting to see whether differences exist between the SOREMP and non-SOREMP sleep periods with respect to the accumulation of SWS. The SWS time, i. e., the time spent in stages 3 and 4, is shown in figure 7b as a function of time elapsed after sleep onset. The dashed and dotted curve and the solid curve represent the SWS accumulation in the SOREMP and non-SOREMP groups, respectively. No significant differences can be noted. Again, we compared our data with those of *Spiegel* [1981] and also with data from *Gaillard* [1977]. The dotted line represents the exponential curve [*Borbely,* 1981] which connects the median values of SWS accumulation calculated from the data of *Spiegel* [1981]. The dashed line represents data from *Gaillard* [1977], measured in young subjects. Our depressive patients show an abnormally low integral duration of SWS time. This is consistent with findings by many others [*Gillin* et al., 1979].

Conclusions

(1) Desynchronization of the temperature rhythm did not occur in our patient group. It cannot, therefore, be a common cause of endogenous depression.

(2) A phase advance of the temperature rhythm is not obvious in our patient group. Thus, a phase disturbance of the temperature rhythm is not likely to be a common cause in depression.

(3) In 7 out of 15 patients it was observed that the circadian modulation in body temperature can be attributed almost completely to the masking influence of the sleep-wake alternation. This finding has not been reported in healthy subjects. It is tempting to speculate that some endogenous depressives suffer from a circadian rhythm disturbance characterized by an extreme flattening of the endogenous temperature oscillation.

Above formulated conclusions can only be preliminary because the possibility on medication artifacts is not yet excluded.

(4) Proper analysis of data on REM sleep production shows that its distribution throughout the night yields no evidence for either of the presently postulated rhythm disturbances in endogenous depression. 20–30 % of the nights in depressives merely show abnormal production of REM sleep in the first hour of sleep.

(5) The decreased SWS production in depressives is a more consistent finding than REM sleep abnormalities.

(6) Conclusions 4 and 5 might prove to be of great importance in future research in depression, because circadian models have recently been proposed in which both some threshold modulation (of which body temperature might be a marker) and SWS production are major variables [*Borbely,* 1981; *Daan and Beersma,* 1982].

Summary

In 27 endogenously depressed patients, continuous recordings of body temperature and motor activity were made and, during some nights, sleep physiology was measured. The data provide no support for either a desynchronization or a phase advance hypothesis. The only chronobiological abnormality encountered in the temperature curves was that some patients showed no circadian temperature oscillation of endogenous origin. The distribution of REM sleep is found to be normal during all nights, except during the first hour of nights with short REM latencies.

References

Åkerstedt, T.; Fröberg, J.E.; Friberg, Y.; Wetterberg, L.: Melatonin excretion, body temperature and subjective arousal during 64 hours of sleep deprivation. Psychoendocrinology *4:* 219–225 (1979).

Atkinson, M.; Kripke, D.F.; Wolf, S.R.: Autorhythmometry in manic depressives. Chronobiologica *2:* 325–335 (1975).

Bemmel, A.L. van; Hoofdakker, R.H. van den: Maintenance of therapeutic effects of total sleep deprivation by limitation of subsequent sleep, a pilot study. Acta psychiat. scand. *63:* 453–462 (1981).

Borbely, A.A.: Sleep regulation: circadian rhythm and homeostasis; in Ganten, Pfaff, Sleep and the autonomic nervous system (Springer, Berlin 1981).

Cahn, H.A.; Polk, G.E.; Huston, P.E.: Age comparison of human day-night physiological differences. Aerospace Med. *39:* 608–610 (1968).

Czeisler, C.A.; Zimmerman, J.C.; Ronda, J.M.; Moore-Ede, M.C.; Weitzman, E.D.: Timing of REM sleep is coupled to the circadian rhythm of body temperature in man. Sleep *2:* 329–346 (1980).

Daan, S.; Beersma, D.G.M.: Circadian gating of human sleep and wakefulness; in Moore-Ede, Mathematical modeling of circadian systems (Raven Press, New York 1983).

Elsenga, S.; Hoofdakker, R.H. van den: Sleep deprivation and clomipramine in endogenous depression; in Popoviciu, Asgian, Dadiu, Sleep 1978 (Karger, Basel 1980).

Gaillard, J.M.: Les tendances générales des stades du sommeil étudiées par ajustements de polynomes orthogonaux. EEG clin. Neurophys. *42:* 847–851 (1977).

Gaillard, J.M.; Martin, L.: Fitting of a parabolic trend to the general component of cumulative occurrence of REM sleep in man; in Levin, Koella, Sleep 1974 (Karger, Basel 1975).

Gillin, J.C.; Duncan, W.; Pettigrew, K.D.; Frankel, B.L.; Snyder, F.: Successful separation of depressed, normal and insomniac subjects by sleep eeg data. Archs gen. Psychiat. *36:* 85–90 (1979).

Hamilton, M.: Development of a rating scale for primary depressive illness. Br. J. Soc. clin. Psychiat. *6:* 278–296 (1967).

Kripke, D.F.; Mullaney, D.J.; Atkinson, M.; Wolf, S.: Circadian rhythm disorders in manic-depressives. Biol. Psychiat. *13:* 335–351 (1978).

Kupfer, D.J.; Foster, F.G.: Interval between onset of sleep and rapid-eye-movement sleep as an indicator of depression. Lancet *1972:* 684–686.

Mulder-Hajonides van der Meulen, W.R.E.H.; Wijnberg, J.R.; Hollander, J.J.; De Diana, I.P.F.; Hoofdakker, R.H. van den: Measurement of subjective sleep quality. 5th Eur. Congr. Sleep-Research, Amsterdam (1980).

Rechtschaffen, A.; Kales, A.: A manual of standardized terminology, techniques and scoring system for sleep stages of human subjects (Bis/Bri, Los Angeles 1968).

Schulz, H.; Lund, R.; Cording, C.; Dirlich, G.: Bimodal distribution of REM sleep latencies in depression. Biol. Psychiat. *14:* 595–600 (1979).

Spiegel, R.: Advances in sleep research, vol. 5; in Weitzman, Sleep and sleeplessness in advanced age (MTP Press, Limited, Lancaster 1981).

Wehr, T.A.; Wirz-Justice, A.: Internal coincidence model for sleep deprivation and depression; in Koella, Sleep 1980 (Karger, Basel 1981).

Wever, R.A.: The circadian system of man. Results of experiments under temporal isolation (Springer, New York 1979).

D.G.M.Beersma, PhD, Department of Biological Psychiatry, Psychiatric University Clinic, Oostersingel 59, NL-9713 EZ Groningen (The Netherlands)

Adv. biol. Psychiat., vol. 11, pp. 128–135 (Karger, Basel 1983)

Chronobiology and Manic Depression
Neuroendocrine and Sleep EEG Parameters

J. Mendlewicz, G. Hoffmann, P. Linkowski, M. Kerkhofs,
J. Golstein, L. Van Haelst, M. L'Hermite, C. Robyn, E. Van Cauter,
V. Weinberg, E. D. Weitzman

Department of Psychiatry, Erasme Hospital, University of Brussels, Belgium

Introduction

Although the hypothalamopituitary axis seems to play a role in the maintenance of circadian rhythms both in animal and man [1], the exact nature of biological clocks remains unclear.

By now it is clear that the pituitary gland constitutes a major link in the neuroendocrine axis in man. Central neurotransmitters regulate the secretion of the hypothalamic neurohormones which in turn may affect brain monoamine metabolism. These neuroendocrine parameters are subjected to circadian variations and they may be implicated in the pathogenesis of periodic psychoses.

Some affective disorders are characterized by an alternation of depressive and manic episodes and by periodic as well as diurnal disturbances in mood and biological functions such as sleep, energy, appetite and sex (evening improvement and morning worsening). These diurnal changes may be related to desynchronization of daynight variation of the mood and drive system. According to this concept, desynchronization may be an important pathophysiological aspect of depression with some biological rhythms following their own free-running, circadian period, deviated from the normal 24-hour period (in general phase advanced).

The study of circadian and ultradian rhytms of biological functions is thus of great importance in psychopathology, in particular, manic depression. According to this desynchronization hypothesis, manic depression may be conceptualized as a 'biological clock' disorder.

Sachar et al. [2] have found that the normal 24-hour pattern of cortisol secretion was disrupted in some depressed patients. There was an increase in the number of secretory episodes, with active secretion during the normal nonsecretory period, and with elevation of all peaks of plasma cortisol throughout the 24 h. The pattern almost returned to normal after the patient recovered. Other workers have previously shown that dexamethasone and insulin-induced hypoglycemia do not suppress cortisol secretion in some depressed patients [3], an observation relating to the same endocrine dysfunction. They postulated the existence of an 'abnormal drive from limbic areas', i.e. there was a central limbic dysfunction in depression. Other studies suggest that these disturbances cannot be explained entirely as a simple stress response, since these abnormalities are present in unanxious patients during sleep and are not corrected after the administration of large doses of sedative medications [4].

In light of the biogenic amine hypothesis of affective illness, recent studies have shown alterations in circadian and seasonal rhythms of various neurotransmitter substances in the plasma of depressed patients [5].

The above arguments led us to examine circadian variations of pituitary-pineal plasma hormone levels in manic depression and to compare the sensitivity of neuroendocrine provocative tests with sleep EEG parameters.

Method

We have investigated pituitary activity in patients suffering from major affective disorders. In this paper, we are reporting results on the 24-hour secretion of prolactin (PRL), thyrotropin (TSH) and melatonin during the depressed phase of manic-depressive illness in subjects diagnosed as bipolar manic-depressives, i.e. patients experiencing both manic and depressive episodes and unipolar depressives, suffering from depression only.

Estimated amplitudes and phases (day and night) of TSH, prolactin and melatonin patterns observed in depressed patients were compared to the estimations obtained for control patterns recorded in healthy volunteers. All patients studied were free of medications for at least one week prior to the investigation and were hospitalized in an inpatient unit for a primary depressive episode severe enough to warrant hospitalization.

Patients were diagnosed as major depressive disorder [6] suffering from bipolar or unipolar depression [7]. Severity of the depressive illness was assessed by the Hamilton Rating Scale [8]. Blood samples were collected every hour during day time and every thirthy minutes during the night. All patients were confined to bed, had normal breakfast, lunch, supper and their nocturnal sleep was not interrupted. Day time sleep was prevented and sleep times were observed by trained nurses. All patients and controls were investigated throughout the calender year.

A detailed description of our methods and results for our pituitary-pineal circadian studies have been published elsewhere [9–11]. We are also presenting preliminary results on

Table I. 24-hour prolactin profiles in unipolar and bipolar patients versus controls

	Normals (n = 14)	Unipolars (n = 10)	Bipolars (n = 8)
24-hour mean (μU/ml)	283 ± 144	351 ± 156	165 ± 62
Wake mean (μU/ml)	235 ± 136	321 ± 158	160 ± 59
Difference between sleep mean and wake mean	+ in 14/14	+ in 8/10	+ in 2/8
Ratio sleep mean/wake mean	1.77 ± 69	1.37 ± 46	1.06 ± 29

REM sleep latency distribution (over 3 consecutive nights) in a new series of depressed patients with major depressive disorders and controls. Comparative data on the performances of the dexamethasone cortisol suppression test [12] and the growth hormone (GH) desimipramine stimulation test [13] are also provided.

Results

The prolactin patterns of all depressive patients as a group (n = 18) showed no significant difference with patterns observed in healthy subjects (n = 6 males). Nevertheless, the mean prolactin level over 24 h was significantly lower in bipolar as compared to unipolar patients. This was mainly due to the absence of sleep-related elevation of PRL in 6 out of 8 bipolar patients (75 %) in whom maximum PRL secretion occurred during wakefulness (phase advanced), whereas maximum PRL concentrations were observed during sleep in all unipolar patients as in normal controls (table I).

The diurnal patterns of *TSH* levels studied in depressed female patients (n = 13) who were not under medication differed greatly from those exhibited by the normal subjects investigated previously (n = 6 males, 10 females). The mean 24-hour TSH level was lower in all depressed patients when compared to normals.

In these patients, the rhythm appears to be desynchronized, no early morning peak being evidenced. In some cases, a maximum occurred before midnight. Higher frequency variation of plasma TSH could also be observed between unipolar and bipolar patients. Furthermore, thyroid function was found to be normal in all patients and controls (table II).

One interesting aspect of the desynchronization hypothesis could be related to the increased incidence of affective (manic and depressive) relapses in spring and autumn when daylight is either longer or shorter. It is

Table II. Nyctohemeral TSH in depression (n = 13)

Unipolar depression	Bipolar depression
Normal thyroid function	Normal thyroid function
Normal basal TSH levels	Normal basal TSH levels
Abnormal circadian TSH rhythm	*Normal circadian TSH rhythm*
Lower 24-hour TSH mean	Normal 24-hour TSH mean
Sleep-wake ratio of TSH is lower	Normal sleep-wake ratio of TSH
Absence of nocturnal rise of TSH	Nocturnal rise of TSH

thus possible that in genetically predisposed subjects, some circadian physiological clock parameters may be desynchronized during these periods. In those susceptible individuals circadian desynchronization may be triggered by infradian seasonal variations and then continue into a free-running cycle.

Melatonin is a pineal hormone particularly sensitive to day-night changes in exposure to light. It is also under central noradrenergic control. Melatonin is thus of great interest when studying cyclic manic-depressive patients. Preliminary data on 24-hour plasma melatonin concentrations are available for 4 female depressed patients before and after treatment and 5 normal controls (males). Secretory episodes are observed during wakefulness in all subjects, but they are of higher magnitude in depressed patients and seem to appear at abnormal times (late afternoon or evening before onset of sleep). Furthermore, the circadian rhythm of melatonin is less apparent in depressed patients. The night/day ratio for melatonin is 1.38 in depressed patients and 2.8 in normals. Nocturnal rise of melatonin is almost absent in 3 of 4 depressed patients who show an elevation of the pituitary hormone during the daytime (phase advanced). Finally, no signficant changes in 24-hour melatonin patterns can be seen in depressed patients after antidepressant treatment and following remission (table III).

It is thus clear that the altered circadian secretion of melatonin in depression is not state-dependent. We are now presenting further data on REM latency and the results of two provocative neuroendocrine tests.

Figures 1 and 2 show the distribution of REM sleep latency (minutes) by night's frequency in 7 non depressed psychiatric controls (4 males and 3 females were 19 to 54 years of age with a mean age of 38) (fig. 1) and 9 depressed patients with major depressive disorders (6 males and 3 females were 25 to 61 years of age with a mean age of 43) (fig. 2). The latter have

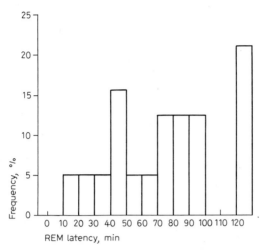

Fig. 1. REM latency distribution in 7 control patients.

Table III. Nyctohemeral melatonin in depression

Nyctohemeral melatonin in depression (n = 4)	Nyctohemeral melatonin in controls (n = 5)
Abnormal or no circadian rhythm	circadian rhythm with nocturnal rise of melatonin
Reduction or absence of nocturnal rise of melatonin	
Average night/day ratio for melatonin = 1.38	night/day ratio for melatonin = 2.80
Secretory episodes throughout the 24-hour span	secretory episodes throughout the 24-hour span

No significant changes in 24-hour melatonin after recovery following antidepressant treatment.

more nights with short REM latencies, illustrating the early occurrence of REM sleep after sleep onset in major depressive disorders [14, 15].

Table IV compares the diagnostic performances of three biological diagnostic parameters. In major depression the higher sensitivity (66 %) is achieved with the REM latency. The specificity and predictive value are excellent for all tests. By using the three biological tests together in the same patients, the sensitivity can be raised up to 78 %, a remarkable value.

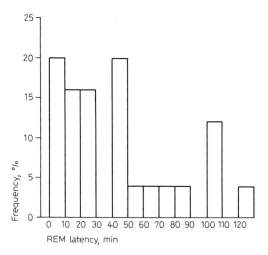

Fig. 2. REM latency distribution in 9 depressed patients with major depressive disorder [6].

Table IV. Diagnostic performances of biological tests in depressed patients with major depressive disorders [6] (n = 9) and controls (n = 7) [according to ref. 16]

	REM latency	Cortisol desamethasone suppression	GH secretion after desimipramine (75 mg i. m.)
Sensitivity, %	66	38	44
Specificity, %	100	86	100
Predictive value, %	100	75	100

Combined sensitivity = 78 %; combined specificity = 100 %; combined predictive value = 100 %.

Alterations in circadian rhythms for plasma pituitary and pineal hormones such as prolactin, TSH and melatonin are present in some depressed patients and it is tempting to hypothesize that these circadian disturbances may be related to the desynchronization phenomenon in manic-depressive illness. This desynchronization may induce primary modifications of circadian rhythms of central catecholaminergic and or serotonergic activity in affective illness, as suggested by the typical altera-tions in 24-hour plasma DBH activity which we have previously described in manic-depressive patients [17]. Moreover, it is possible that cholinergic-adrenergic interactions are also of importance as it has been postulated for REM sleep latency [18] and for the DST [19]. More fruitful hypotheses may be formulated in terms of infradian, ultradian or circadian variation in specific brain receptor sensitivity or more complex behavioral modulation through endogenous neuropeptide substances.

The brain distribution of other releasing factors and peptides has not yet been reported and when the brain effects of hypothalamic hormones and peptides will be further elucidated, the clinical conditions in which their actions are investigated may be better understood. Nevertheless, the chronobiological studies described above combining neurophysiological and neuroendocrine evaluation over long periods of time in the study of abnormal behavior are most promising and may enable us to better understand cyclical alterations of hypothalamic and pituitary functions in man, although it is still premature to draw firm conclusions form the neuroendocrine abnormalities as to the specific nature of the underlying neurotransmitter or neuropeptide disturbances in psychopathology. A combination strategy using simultaneous neuroendocrine and sleep EEG evaluations may nevertheless provide us with sensitive, specific and reliable biological tools for the diagnosis and treatment of affective disorders.

References

1   Richter, C. P.: Abnormal but regular cycles in behavior and metabolism in rats and catatonic-schizophrenics; in Reiss, Psychoneuroendocrinology, pp. 168–181 (Grune & Stratton, New York 1958).

2   Sachar, E. J.; Hellman, L.; Fukushima, D. K.: Cortisol production in depressive illness. Archs gen. Psychiat. *23:* 289–298 (1970).

3   Carroll, B. J.: Hypothalamic-pituitary function in depressive illness. Insensitivity to hypoglycaemia. Br. med. J. *iii:* 27–28 (1969).

4   Stokes, P. E.: Studies on the control of adrenocortical function in depression; in Williams, Katz, Shiled, Recent advances in the psychobiology of depressive illnesses, pp. 199–220, Washington D. C., (US DEHW, 1972).

5   Riederer, P.; Birkmayer, W.; Neumayer, E.; Ambrozi, L.; Linauer, W.: The daily rhythm of HVA, VMA, (VA) and 5HIAA in depression syndrome. J. neural Transm. *35:* 23–45 (1974).

6   Spitzer, R. L.; Endicott, J.; Robins, E.: Research diagnostic criteria. Archs gen. Psychiat. *35:* 773–782 (1978).

7   Mendlewicz, J.; Fleiss, J. L.: Linkage studies with X-chromosome markers in bipolar (manic-depressive) and unipolar (depressive) illness. Biol. Psychiat. *2:* 1044 (1974).

8   Hamilton, M. A.: A rating scale for depression. J. Neurol. Neurosurg. Psychiat. *23:* 56 (1960).

9   Mendlewicz, J.; Van Cauter, E.; Linkowksi, P.; L'Hermite, M.; Robyn, C.: The 24-hour profile of prolactin in depression. Life Sci. *27:* 2015–2024 (1980).

10   Golstein, J.; Van Cauter, E.; Linkowski, P.; Vanhaelst, L.; Mendlewicz, J.: Thyrotrophin nyctohemeral pattern in primary depression. Differences between unipolar and bipolar women. Life Sci. *27:* 1695–1704 (1980).

11   Mendlewicz, J.; Branchey, L.; Weinberg, U.; Branchey, M.; Linkowski, P.; Weitzman, E. D.: The 24-hour pattern of plasma melatonin in depressed patients before and after treatment. Commun. Psychopharmacol. *4:* 49–55 (1980).

12   Carroll, B. J.; Schroeder, K.; Mukhopadhyay, S.; Greden, J. F.; Feinberg, M.; Ritche, J.; Tarika, J.: Plasma dexamethasone concentrations and cortisol supression response in patients with endogenous depression. J. clin. Endocr. Metab. *51:* 433–437 (1980).

13   Laakmann, G.: Neuroendocrinological findings in affective disorders after administration of antidepressants. Adv. Biol. Psychiat., vol. 5, pp. 67–84 (Karger, Basel 1980).

14   Schulz, H.; Lund, R.; Cording, C.; Dirlich, G.: Bimodal distribution of REM sleep latencies in depression. Biol. Psychiat. *14:* 595–600 (1979).

15   Coble, P. A.; Kupfer, D. J.; Shaw, D. H.: Distribution of REM latency in depression. Biol. Psychiat. *17:* 453–466 (1981).

16   Carroll, B. J.: Implications of biological research for the diagnosis of depression; in Mendlewicz, New advances in the diagnosis and treatment of depressive illness, pp. 85–107 (1980).

17   Van Cauter, E.; Mendlewicz, J.: 24-hour dopamine-beta-hydroxylase pattern. A possible biological index of manic-depression. Life Sci. *22:* 147–155 (1978).

18   Sitaram, N.; Nornberger, J. I.; Elliot, J. R.; Gershon, S.; Christian Gillin, J.: Faster cholinergic REM sleep induction in euthymic patients with primary affective illness. Science *208:* 200–201 (1980).

19   Carroll, B. J.; Greden, J. F.; Rubin, R. T.; Haskett, R. F.; Feinberg, M.; Schteingart, D.: Neurotransmitter mechanism of neuroendocrine disturbance in depression. Acta endocr., Copenh., suppl. 220, p. 14 (1978).

J. Mendlewicz, MD, PhD, Department of Psychiatry, Erasme Hospital, University of Brussels, B-1070 Brussels (Belgium)

Adv. biol. Psychiat., vol. 11, pp. 136–149 (Karger, Basel 1983)

Biological Rhythms in Man under Non-Entrained Conditions and Chronotherapy for Delayed Sleep Phase Insomnia

Elliot D. Weitzman

Institute of Chronobiology, New York Hospital-Cornell Medical Center, Westchester Division and Cornell University Medical College, White Plains, N.Y., USA

Recognition of the laws governing biological rhythm functions in man has greatly increased our understanding of the physiology of human sleep. Based on continuous recordings of electroencephalographic, electromyographic, and eye movement activity, and measurements of heart rate, blood pressure, hormones and respiration, we now know what patterns of activity normally occur during sleeping and waking hours. Recent studies in our laboratory have uncovered changes in body temperature, secretion of plasma and urinary hormones, alertness, performance efficiency, and mood which also correlate with sleep-wake patterns.

It is well known that experimentally altering 'zeitgebers' (time cues) can change the lawful relationships between chronobiological rhythms. However, numerous studies show that the new cycles which develop during non-entrained free-running conditions also follow consistent and lawful patterns, but with significant intersubject variability. These individual differences are of considerable interest. They suggest that even under everyday conditions, certain people experience and internal shifts of their chronobiological rhythms which produce specific sleep and arousal disorders.

This concept is supported by recent studies in a group of patients with the newly identified syndrome, delayed sleep phase insomnia. We find that progressively delaying the time at which they go to sleep can effectively reset these patients' biological rhythms, to restore their normal sleep patterns.

As this result suggests, our knowledge of chronobiology can significantly improve the evaluation and treatment of sleep-wake abnormalities in man. The brief discussion which follows describes continuing research in our laboratory (Laboratory of Human Chronophysiology) focusing on the timing, length, sequencing, and internal organization of biological rhythms during entrained and free-running conditions. Our work and that of other investigators is rapidly expanding the interface between basic research in chronobiology and clinical therapy of human sleep-wake disorders.

Studies in Normal Man during Non-Entrained Conditions

We have constructed a specially designed Laboratory of Human Chronophysiology in which subjects can live for many weeks under conditions of temporal isolation. Unlike other research projects which totally isolate subjects from human contact, we provide frequent social communication. This also permits us to make biological measurements and psychological observations that are not possible in other laboratories. In addition, we have developed techniques for obtaining plasma samples from our subjects at approximately 20-min intervals, so that we can analyze temporal patterns of hormone secretion. Using this approach, we have discovered important relationships between hormonal blood concentrations, sleep, and sleep stages [*Weitzman* et al., 1966, 1971, 1975; *Weitzman,* 1976; *Hellman* et al., 1970].

Period Length
In many published studies, biological rhythms and hormone secretion are measured only during entrained 24-hour sessions. Our current work examines important changes that occur when subjects are not entrained to external time cues. We have confirmed earlier reports that biological rhythms of human beings free-run at period lengths greater than 24 h, usually approximating 25 h. In our group of 10 normal men, individual subjects varied, but many spontaneously developed 'long' biologic days greater than 35 h, which often alternated with 'short' days of approximately 25 h.

Length of Sleep
During free-running, the length of sleep was correlated with the phase of the circadian core (rectal) body temperature rhythm, and not with the duration of prior wakefulness (fig. 1). We found that long sleep episodes of 12–18 h occurred when subjects chose to go to sleep at or near the peak of the averaged circadian body temperature cycle. Shorter sleep episode

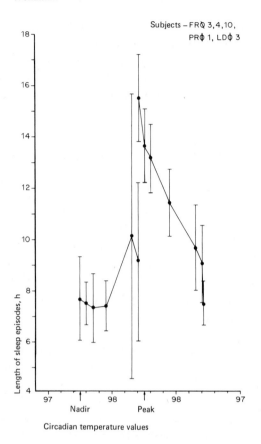

Fig. 1. Relationship between mean (± SD) sleep duration and temperature for 5 subjects during free-running. The temperature values chosen were derived an enduced circadian temperature curve, each value representing sequential 30° of circadian phase.

durations of 6–8 h occurred at the nadir [*Weitzman* et al., 1979; *Czeisler,* 1978; *Czeisler* et al., 1980 b, 1981].

REM Sleep

Free-running conditions also produced a phase advance of REM sleep to an earlier time during sleep. That is, REM latency shortened significantly, often to less than 10 min after sleep onset, with an associated increase in REM amounts during the first 3 h of sleep. However, the total REM amount and percent for an entire sleep episode remained constant [*Weitzman* et al., 1980].

Just as we found for the length of sleep episodes, the timing and amount of REM sleep following sleep onset also was correlated with specific phases of the circadian temperature cycle [*Czeisler* et al., 1980c]. Studies that were not performed in conditions of temporal isolation, but which allowed unrestricted sleep in normal subjects who were awake for different lengths of time prior to sleep, showed a similar circadian rhythm of sleep episode duration and a strong correlation between REM sleep and body temperature [*Åkerstedt and Gillberg,* 1981]. These data strongly suggest that certain sleep processes in the brain are influenced by an underlying endogenous biological rhythm oscillator, and not by the sleep process itself.

In contrast to REM sleep, stages 3 and 4 sleep did not phase shift during free-running conditions. Even for long sleep periods greater than 10 h, stages 3 and 4 recurred after 14–16 h of sleep. There also were no differences in the REM-non-REM cycle length during entrained and free-running conditions. We propose that stages 3 and 4 are not primarily dependent on the total duration of sleep or the length of prior waking, but are related to the length of prior elapsed time [*Weitzman* et al., 1980].

Body Temperature

Under entrainment, core temperature typically showed only a small decrease approximately 3 h before sleep onset, and then dropped sharply (1–2°F) following sleep onset. At the end of the sleep episode, temperature rose sharply.

During free-running, however, temperature developed an approximately 25-hour rhythm, but with a 6- to 8-hour advance of the falling phase. That is, temperature began to decrease 6–8 h prior to sleep onset and at the time of choosing sleep, the body temperature was approaching the lowest value of the circadian rhythm, with an additional small drop (0.5–1.0°F) occurring just after sleep onset. This added drop in body temperature was especially prominent at the onset of the long sleep episodes, when the immediately preceding core temperature was high [*Weitzman* et al., 1981b].

Plasma Cortisol and Growth Hormone

We were successful in obtaining 20-min interval plasma samples for the entire study from 9 of our subjects (aged 22–51 years), who were studied during 5 days of entrainment, followed by longer periods of free-running. Analyses of these samples showed a very stable and consistent pattern of cortisol and growth hormone secretion, both between subjects and for each individual subject (fig. 2 a, b).

There was no significant difference in the amount, rate, or number of cortisol and growth hormone secretory episodes during 24 h under entrained or free-running conditions. However, the free-running circadian cortisol secretion curve showed two distinct components. One component had a 6- to 8-hour phase advance relative to sleep onset, much like the advance in REM sleep and the nadir of the body temperature curve. The second component, which clearly followed sleep onset, was characterized by a distinct inhibition of cortisol secretion during the first 2–3 h of sleep, interrupting a rising phase of the hormonal curve. Another time-locked episode of cortisol secretion occurred just following waking [*Weitzman* et al., 1979, 1980, 1981c].

In contrast, the temporal pattern of growth hormone secretion was directly related to sleep onset, during both entrained and free-running conditions. A major episode of hormonal secretion occurred within the first 2 h after sleep onset for almost all sleep episodes, but not at the time of waking [*Weitzman* et al., 1979, 1980]. This demonstrated an inverse relationship between cortisol and growth hormone both at sleep onset and at waking [*Weitzman* et al., 1981c].

All of these findings suggest that specific brain mechanisms simultaneously control the yoked release of ACTH-cortisol and the inhibition of growth hormone secretion, or at other times, the simultaneous inhibition of cortisol secretion and release of growth hormone. During 'activation' at the time of waking, there is inhibition of growth hormone and secretion of cortisol. During stages 3 and 4 sleep, immediately following sleep onset, there is partial inhibition of ACTH-cortisol and a major secretion of growth hormone [*Weitzman* et al., 1981b].

Performance, Alertness, and Mood

Because our experimental setting permits social communication, we also have been able to study performance and subjective alertness during entrained and free-running conditions. Measurements were taken in 8 subjects during self-selected wake times only, thereby eliminating the confounding influence of sleep deprivation and sleep interruptions. All subjects completed self-reports at frequent intervals, by marking continuous vertical scales ranging from 'very alert' to 'sleepy'. Subjects also received performance tests at waketime, and prior to meals, urinations, and bedtime. For 7 subjects, the performance task consisted of the speed of

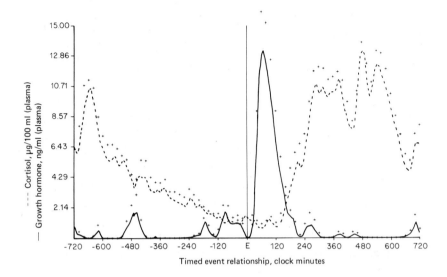

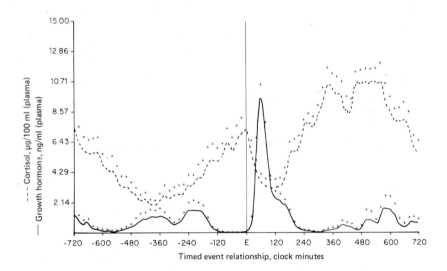

Fig. 2. a Graph of timed event relationship (mean ± SEM) of plasma cortisol (μg/100 ml) for subject AE (4 sleep-wake cycles) at sleep onset (E) for all sleep episodes during entrainment. *b* Graph of timed event relationship (mean ± SEM) of plasma growth hormone (ng/ml) for subject AE at sleep onset for all sleep episodes during free-running sleep.

simply sorting 96 playing cards into red and black piles. The performance measure was sorting time. The remaining subject performed a more complex visual-motor test that involved tracking a target with a electronic rod. The performance measure was the accuracy of tracking during a fixed time interval.

During entrained waking periods, we found that a gradual increase in temperature was associated with a progressive rise in subjective alertness and an increase in performance efficiency. Subjective alertness fell at the end of the day, but performance remained stable throughout.

During free-running, the pattern was reversed. Performance efficiency remained stable throughout most of the day, but showed a rapid decrement as temperature and subjective alertness reached their nadir prior to bedtime. In both entrained and free-running conditions, performance efficiency was more closely related to the temperature cycle than it was to subjective alertness. Performance was worst at the temperature nadir and best at the temperature peak.

Some subjects also completed mood scales. During entrainment, we found an increase in positive mood states throughout the day, correlated with an increase in body temperature, performance efficiency, and subjective alertness. During free-running conditions, moods of happiness and relaxation continued to increase in the subjects' morning hours, and to level off thereafter. On the other hand, 'enthusiasm', 'concentration', and 'energy' during free-running were closely related to the pattern of body temperature and subjective alertness, increasing in the morning and gradually declining throughout the rest of the waking day [*Zimmerman* et al., 1981].

Clinical Applications: Delayed Sleep Phase Syndrome

Our studies demonstrate that the phase of endogenous circadian rhythms, rather than the sleep-wake cycle, is a major determinant of the timing of sleep onset, sleep length, REM sleep, cortisol secretion, performance, alertness, and mood. What makes these findings so important is their direct application to the diagnosis and treatment of affective disorders and clinical sleep-wake abnormalities. *Wehr* et al. [1979], for example, reported that phase advancing the sleep time in several patients with bipolar manic-depressive illness repeatedly produced an immediate switch out of depression. REM deprivation [*Vogel* et al., 1975] and total sleep deprivation [*Rudolf* et al., 1977] can achieve similar results. Based on evidence that an advance in REM sleep develops during depressive illness, *Vogel* et al. [1980] proposed a chronobiological explanation for the therapeutic effectiveness of REM deprivation.

Laboratory studies of phase advances in REM sleep after transmeridian rapid flights [*Weitzman* et al., 1970; *Klein* et al., 1977; *Hume,* 1980] demonstrate the importance of biological rhythm functions in sleep disturbances as well. Investigation of patients with frequently changing sleep-wake schedules also shows that disruption of normal rhythms disrupts and shortens sleep periods. Subjects also experience impaired performance and alertness, and suffer from excessive sleepiness alternating with periods of arousal, often at inconvenient and inappropriate times of day [*Rentos and Shephard,* 1976].

These findings, coupled with data from physiological studies of temperature and hormonal secretion, suggest that the brain oscillators which control sleep-wake cycles in man can become desynchronized under certain social or environmental conditions. This hypothesis has gained considerable support from our recent investigations of delayed sleep phase insomnia.

During a 3-year period in which we studied 450 patients whose primary complaint fit the diagnostic classification of 'insomnias' it became clear to us that a subgroup of patients showed major symptoms that were distinguishable from other forms of insomnia. We identified 30 patients whose characteristic complaint was a chronic inability to fall asleep at a desired clock time required to meet work or study schedules, and a great difficulty in morning awakening [*Weitzman* et al., 1981a].

Typically these subjects showed a long sleep latency and were unable to fall asleep until 2–6 a.m. (fig. 3). However, on weekends, holidays and vacations, when they were not required to maintain a strict schedule, they slept for a normal length of time without difficulty, and awakened spontaneously, feeling refreshed, but, of course, at a later hour. Polysomnographic recordings in the sleep laboratory indicated that sleep length and internal organization was normal when these patients were permitted to choose their sleep time (usually 4–5 a.m. to noon–1 p.m.). However, when sleep is attempted earlier in the night, a long latency occurred before sleep onset.

Patients such as these are usually diagnosed as having 'sleep onset insomnia', and are often treated with hypnotic drugs, alcohol, behavior modification, sleep hypnosis, psychotherapy, and other remedies – all of

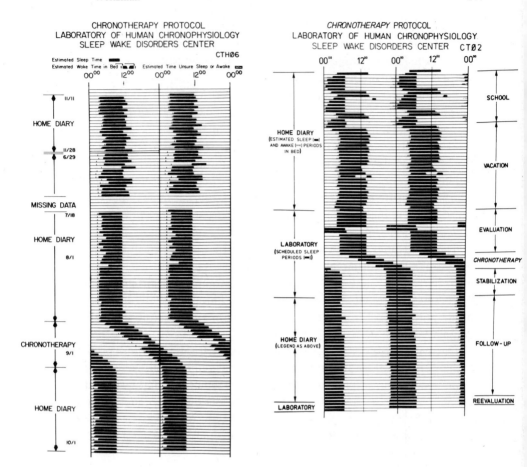

Fig. 3. Daily sleep-wake pattern of 2 patients with diagnosis of delayed sleep phase syndrome before and after chronotherapy. Pattern is displayed as 'double plot' to demonstrate phase shift beyond the 24-hour period.

them generally ineffective. Attempts to phase advance the time of going to sleep to an earlier time also usually fails in these patients.

Chronotherapy

We have proposed a new approach to treating delayed sleep phase syndrome, which successfully eliminates insomnia, without drugs [*Weitz-*

man et al., 1981a; *Czeisler* et al., 1981]. Using a progressive phase delay of the sleep time – that is, delaying the time of going to sleep by 3 h each day, for a 27-hour sleep-wake cycle – we can reset the patient's sleep time to occur at a socially acceptable hour (fig. 3).

This single 5- to 6-day treatment was tested in 7 patients with a 4- to 15-year history of delayed sleep phase insomnia. All experience a lasting resolution of their symptoms, confirmed by long-term self-reports during follow-up periods ranging from 42 to 910 days (average 260 days), and by objective polygraphic recordings before and after treatment. The average sleep onset shifted from 4:50 a.m. before chronotherapy, to 12:20 a.m. afterwards, with no reduction in sleep efficiency. As a result of this significant improvement, all patients were able to end a long-term dependence on hypnotic drugs.

Phase-Advance Shifts

These dramatic results support our hypothesis that patients with delayed sleep phase insomnia have a diminished capacity to make phase-advance shifts in their sleep-wake cycle. From our studies in free-running conditions, we know that normal human subjects develop a sleep-wake cycle approximating 25 h. This indicates that the normal internal biologic clock runs a little slower than its mechanical or geophysical counterparts. Consequently, for human circadian rhythms to be successfully entrained to a 24-hour day, the biological clock must be actively phase-advanced by an average of 1 h each day.

When the light-dark cycle and other events are experimentally controlled, normal subjects can be entrained to period lengths ranging from about 23–27 h. We hypothesize that delayed sleep phase syndrome patients have an abnormality of this 'normal range of entrainment'. Although they can successfully entrain their sleep-wake times to occur at about the same clock hours daily, they lack sufficient phase-advancing capacity to shift sleep time to earlier clock hours. Because synchronizing cues from the environment are only weakly able to prevent their sleep episodes from drifting progressively later into the afternoon, these subjects have considerable difficulty advancing to achieve resynchronization.

The biological mechanism underlying this problem is not known, but we believe it may be related to the phase-response curve (PRC) [*Weitzman* et al., 1981a; *Czeisler* et al., 1981]. PRCs have been measured in many mammalian, submammalian, and plant species by applying an effective stimulus such as light, to a non-entrained organism at different time points

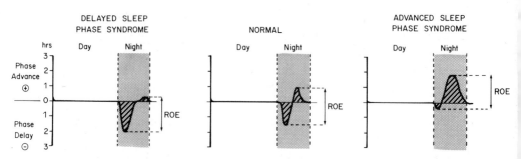

Fig. 4. Hypothetical phase response curves and range of entrainment (ROE) for two chronobiological disorders. Patients with delayed sleep phase could have abnormally small *phase advance* capability whereas those with an advanced sleep phase could have an abnormally small phase delay capability.

in the circadian cycle, and then observing the amount and direction of a phase-shift response [*Bunning,* 1973; *Aschoff* et al., 1975].

Phase changes of the sleep-wake cycle in man may be induced by wakefulness during the usual sleep episode. Therefore, early awakening produces a phase advance of the sleep period on the following night, whereas late retiring produces a phase delay. For normal subjects, this biphasic form of the PRC maintains entrainment to environmental timed stimuli, such as the morning alarm clock, even when these stimuli are shifted from night to night. For subjects with delayed sleep phase syndrome, however, the phase-advance portion of the PRC may be much less prominent (fig. 4). Whenever bedtime occurs later than usual, the phase-delay mechanism is activated, but the compensatory phase advance mechanism is weak and fails to effectively reset the sleep time. The net result is a shift of sleep to a later time [*Weitzman* et al., 1981a].

Based on this analysis, we recognized that it is not sufficient to help delayed sleep phase syndrome patients *achieve* a more desirable phase position. They would also need help to *maintain* it. Since chronotherapy may not change underlying abnormalities in the circadian pacemakers, we recognized that after even minor temporary shifts of the sleep-wake schedule, due to late parties on weekends or travel to a westward time zone, for example, these patients will have great difficulty or be unable to return to their desired phase position. We therefore recommend that patients avoid relapses by strictly maintaining a regular sleep-wake schedule.

The ability of our patients to maintain their new, previously unattainable sleep schedules for months and years following this simple treatment, refutes suggestions that the intrusive thinking is causing the inability of fall asleep. The relationship of abnormal personality characteristics and other psychopathology to the altered PRC clearly needs further study. Our research on biological rhythms points to new and effective non-drug treatment for some types of insomnia, and possibly for sleep-wake rhythm disorders related to aging, neuroendocrine dysfunctions, and other endogenously controlled biological functions [*Weitzman* et al., 1981a].

Summary

Studies of subjects living under entrained and non-entrained free-running conditions, demonstrate a linkage between circadian rhythms of cortisol secretion, body temperature, and REM sleep, which shift relative to sleep onset, and a corresponding linkage between growth hormone secretion and non-REM sleep, which remain tied to sleep onset. We hypothesize that sleep-wake disorders in man may reflect disruptions in the lawful relationships between these chronobiological rhythms. This hypothesis is supported by studies in patients with delayed sleep phase insomnia, a new syndrome involving sleep-onset insomnia and difficult morning awakening. Nondrug chronotherapy effectively eliminated insomnia in all patients tested.

References

Åkerstedt, T.; Gillberg, M.: The circadian pattern of unrestricted sleep and its relation to body temperature, hormones and alertness. Proc. 1979 ONR/NIOSH Symp. variation in work-sleep schedules: effects on healt and performance. Adv. Sleep Res. *6* (in press 1981).

Aschoff, J.; Hoffmann, K.; Pohl, H. et al.: Re-entrainment of ciradian rhythms after phase-shifts of the zeitgeber. Chronobiologia *2:* 23–78 (1975).

Bunning, E.: The physiological clock; 3rd ed. (Springer, New York 1973).

Czeisler, C. A.: Human circadian physiology: internal organization of temperature, sleep-wake and neuroendocrine function in an environment free of time cues; PhD dissertation, Stanford University (1978).

Czeisler, C. A.; Richardson, G. S.; Coleman, R. et al.: Chronotherapy: Resetting the circadian clock of patients with delayed sleep phase insomnia. Sleep *4:* 1–21 (1981).

Czeisler, C. A.; Weitzman, E. D.; Moore-Ede, M. C.; Zimmerman, J. C.; Knauer, R. S.: Human sleep: its duration and organization depend on its circadian phase. Science *210:* 1264–1267 (1980a).

Czeisler, C. A.; Weitzman, E. D.; Moore-Ede, M. C.; Kronauer, R. E.; Zimmerman, J. C.; Campbell, C.: Human sleep: its duration and structure depend on the interaction of two separate circadian oscillators (Abstract). Sleep Res. *9* (in press, 1980b).

Czeisler, C. A.; Zimmerman, J. C.; Ronda, J. M.; Moore-Ede, M. C.; Weitzman, E. D.: Timing of REM sleep is coupled to the circadian rhythm of body temperature in man. Sleep 2: 329–346 (1980c).

Hellman, L.; Weitzman, E. D.; Roffwarg, H.; Fukushima, D. K.; Yoshida, K.; Gallagher, T. F.: Cortisol is secreted episodically in Cushing's syndrome. J. clin. Endocr. Metab. 30: 686–689 (1970).

Hume, K. I.: Sleep adaptation after phase shifts of the sleep-wakefulness rhythm in man. Sleep 2: 417–435 (1980).

Klein, K. E.; Hermann, H.; Kuklinski, P.; Wegmann, H.-M.: Circadian performance rhythms: experimental studies in air operation; in Mackie, Vigilance: theory, operational performance and physiological correlates, pp. 117–132 (Plenum Press, New York 1977).

Rentos, P. G.; Shephard, R. D.: Shift work and health: a symposium (National Institute for Occupational Safety and Health, Office of Extramural Activities, Washington 1976).

Rudolf, G. A. E.; Schilgen, B.; Tolle, R.: Anti-depressive Behandlung mittels Schlafentzug. Nervenarzt 48: 1–11 (1977).

Vogel, G. W.; Thurmond, A.; Gibbons, P.; Sloan, K.; Boyd, M.; Walker, M.: REM sleep reduction effects on depression syndromes. Archs gen. Psychiat. 32: 765–777 (1975).

Vogel, G. W.; Vogel, F.; McAbee, R. S.; Thurmond, A. J.: Improvement of depression by REM sleep deprivation. Archs gen. Psychiat. 37: 247–253 (1980).

Wehr, T.; Wirz-Justice, A.; Goodwin, R. K.; Duncan, W.; Gillin, J. C.: Phase advance of the circadian sleep-wake cycle as an anti-depressant. Science 206: 710–711 (1979).

Weitzman, E. D.: Circadian rhythms and episodic hormone secretion in man. A. Rev. Med. 27: 225–243 (1976).

Weitzman, E. D.; Boyar, R. M.; Kapen, S.; Hellman, L.: The relationships of sleep and sleep stages to neuroendocrine secretion and biological rhythms in man. Recent Prog. Horm. Res. 31: 399–440 (1975).

Weitzman, E. D.; Czeisler, C. A.; Coleman, R. M.; Spielman, A. J.; Zimmerman, J. C.; Dement, W.: Delayed sleep phase syndrome. Archs gen. Psychiat. 38: 737–746 (1981a).

Weitzman, E. D.; Czeisler, C. A.; Moore-Ede, M.: Sleep-wake, neuroendocrine and body temperature circadian rhythms under entrained and non-entrained (free-running) conditions in man; in Suda, Hayaishi, Nakagawa, Biological rhythms and their central mechanism, pp. 199–227 (Elsevier/North Holland, New York 1979).

Weitzman, E. D.; Czeisler, C. A.; Zimmerman, J. C.; Moore-Ede, M. C.: Biological rhythms in man: relationship of sleep-wake, cortisol, growth hormone and temperature during temporal isolation; in Martin, Reichlin, Bick, Neurosecretion and brain peptides, pp. 475–496 (Raven Press, New York 1981b).

Weitzman, E. D.; Czeisler, C. A.; Zimmerman, J. C.; Ronda, J. M.: Timing of REM and stages 3 + 4 sleep during temporal isolation in man. Sleep 2: 391–407 (1980).

Weitzman, E. D.; Czeisler, C. A.; Zimmerman, J. C.; Ronda, J. M.: Temporal organization of cortisol and growth hormone secretion in entrained and nonentrained man. 12th World Congress of Neurology, Kyoto (in press, 1981c).

Weitzman, E. D.; Fukushima, D.; Nogeire, C.; Roffwarg, H.; Gallagher, T. F.; Hellman, L.: The twenty-four hour pattern of the episodic secretion of cortisol in normal subjects. J. clin. Endocr. Metab. 33: 14–22 (1971).

Weitzman, E. D.; Kripke, D.; Goldmacher, D.; McGregor, P.; Nogeire, C.: Acute reversal of the sleep-waking cycle in man. Archs Neurol., Chicago 22: 483–489 (1970).

Weitzman, E.D.; Schaumburg, H.; Fishbein, W.: Plasma 17-hydroxycorticosteroid levels during sleep in man. J. clin. Endocr. Metab. *26:* 121–127 (1966).

Zimmerman, J.C.; Czeisler, C.A.; Weitzman, E.D.: Chronobiology of performance and moods during temporal isolation in humans. Adv. Sleep Res. *6* (in press, 1981).

E. D. Weitzman, MD, Institute of Chronobiology, New York Hospital-Cornell Medical Center, Westchester Division and Cornell University Medical College, White Plains, NY 10605 (USA)